The Honey Diet

I dedicate this book to my wife Theresa.

Mike McInnes

The Honey Diet

CORONET

First published in Great Britain in 2014 by Coronet
An imprint of Hodder & Stoughton
An Hachette UK company

1

A CIP catalogue record for this title is
available from the British Library

Typeset in Sabon MT by Palimpsest Book Production Limited,
Falkirk, Stirlingshire
Printed and bound by Clays Ltd, St Ives plc

ISBN 9781444775907

Hodder & Stoughton policy is to use papers that are natural, renewable
and recyclable products and made from wood grown in sustainable
forests. The logging and manufacturing processes are expected to
conform to the environmental regulations of the country of origin.

Hodder & Stoughton Ltd
338 Euston Road
London NW1 3BH
www.hodder.co.uk

CONTENTS

INTRODUCTION

If you have always battled with your weight or you are just beginning to thicken a bit around the middle, bottom or thighs, you will know that slimming is not easy. In fact, it is extremely difficult.

There is something so frustrating about the fact that the minute you think about going on a diet, or even just try to cut back on treats and goodies, you will become strangely obsessed with food.

It is confounding, and makes losing weight feel like a mammoth task.

But I have discovered the reason – and the solution.

There is no need for anyone to go on a drastic calorie-counted diet. You DEFINITELY don't want to be stocking up on diet products and you don't have to subject yourself to a life of bitter, gritty brown foods with no sweetness.

The Honey Diet is refreshingly simple: it is all about good, healthy eating, with honey at its heart.

This book is backed by strong science. As a scientist myself, I have spent decades researching this subject and I am convinced that the root of our big obesity problem is the fact that most of us eat far too much sugar and junk food. Even when we think we are eating 'healthy' low-fat foods, they will very often be packed with hidden sugars or white flour (which the body swiftly converts to sugar).

Many of us inadvertently make poor food choices all day long. You might start your day with sweetened cereal for breakfast (your bowl of Frosties contains 3½ teaspoons sugar), nibble on a couple of biscuits with your morning coffee (1 teaspoon sugar in each), down a fizzy drink (5 to 6 teaspoons) with your white bread sandwich at lunchtime, grab a bar of chocolate (10 teaspoons) to stave off the mid-afternoon snoozes, then sit down to a big bowl of white pasta with a large glass of wine in the evening.

With a perfectly normal modern diet like this, there's a real possibility that your blood sugar levels will bubble away on maximum all day long.

The body's best method of dealing with this sugar overload is to release quantities of a hormone called insulin which directs excess sugar out of the blood and into the fat cells for storage.

This, quite simply, is how sugar makes us fat.

But I believe this abundance of sugar in our diets has far more sinister consequences for our health than its impact on our weight.

The source of the problem is an intricate pumping mechanism that controls and delivers fuel to the neurones – the thinking cells in the brain. For every neurone, there are ten or more special 'feeder cells', called 'glial cells', each of which houses a tiny pump. Scientists call this system the 'cerebral glucose pump', but I call it the iPump.

This highly intelligent brain pump has an incredibly important job. It ensures a steady and very carefully monitored supply of fuel to the neurones.

If the iPump detects too much sugar in the blood – a saturation that could be dangerous for the brain's delicate tissues – it trips a switch (just like the power breaker in an electric cable). This closes the iPump valves, temporarily cutting back the fuel supply to the neurones to an absolute minimum.

This clever mechanism evolved to protect the brain from sugar overload. It allows just enough fuel through for the brain cells to continue to function, without any risk of catastrophic sugar overload.

In the distant past, when times were hard and sugar feasts were few and far between, the iPump would rarely close off, and, if it did, would only remain closed for a very short time. But today, there's sugar in virtually everything we consume, and this means that the pump can be switched to emergency mode for VERY long periods of time.

And there's where we come unstuck. When the valve is partially closed, the iPump won't allow enough fuel through for the brain to operate at full capacity, or anything like it. It is on emergency measures only.

If this goes on for more than around 15 minutes, the brain starts to get hungry and that makes it stressed. In desperation, it will send out a cocktail of chemical messages to drum up glucose from any other possible sources, driving us to eat more and more and more.

If we respond to these cravings and continue to eat (as so many of us do), blood sugar levels will stay high and the iPump could end up being switched to emergency mode for days, weeks . . . even years.

The more we eat, the longer the iPump stays off, and the hungrier and more stressed our brain becomes.

I am convinced that millions of people are walking around with hungry stressed brains the whole time. You might notice this as cravings – particularly for sweet foods – because sugar is what the brain needs. This isn't a gentle hint. The demands from your brain are so strong that even the most resolute will-power CANNOT deny them. This is why it's so hard to stop at one biscuit, one square of chocolate, or one handful of popcorn, and why some people can eat and eat and eat and become so obese they need mechanical cranes to lift them out of bed.

Memory lapses and wavers in concentration could be a sign that your brain is struggling to cope without enough fuel.

The chemicals and hormones your hungry brain sends out in its desperate attempts to get the fuel it needs are really very bad for us. This is the chemical cascade that leads to heart disease, dementia, depression, even some cancers.

There have been numerous studies over the years confirming a link between obesity and ill-health and the iPump is one clear reason why.

But the good news is that there is a quick and easy way to break this vicious cycle – and honey holds the key.

It is sugar and refined white carbohydrates that cause the iPump system to malfunction, but honey behaves completely differently in the body. It is uniquely designed to provide the brain with the fuel it needs without compromising the iPump, and without causing any stress-related problems.

By simply switching from sugar to honey in your diet, you will be doing enough to stop your cravings for bad sugars, feed your poor hungry, stressed brain, reset your iPump, and get your body back to functioning exactly as it should.

If you've picked up this book because you want to lose weight, you should know that the other good reason why you're getting fat and the diets don't seem to be working is very likely to be because you're not sleeping properly, or not sleeping enough, and – again – that's because of the sugar and junk food in your diet. Honey can help.

If your iPump gets tripped during the night (or if it just ends up staying tripped long term), your brain will be hungry and stress hormones will be washing around your body. Their levels might not be high enough to keep you awake, but they could certainly be responsible for a fitful and unsatisfying night's sleep. Throughout the night, when your body is supposed to be recovering and repairing damaged tissues, those stress chemicals will be wreaking havoc instead.

But if your iPump is allowed to work properly, and you sleep well, your body can get busy with its nightly repair process and your brain can effectively reboot itself ready for the day ahead. If done properly, with the iPump working as it should, this night-time process burns body fat – a LOT of body fat.

Sleep badly, and the repair process – and fat burning – just doesn't happen.

Want a simple solution? My research has shown that you can reset your iPump, and ensure a great night's fat-burning sleep, by taking 50g (around 2 tablespoons) of honey before you go to bed.

This works because, unlike any other sugar, honey is uniquely formulated to replenish the brain's fuel reserves, keeping the brain well supplied throughout the night, without disrupting the delicate iPump.

So my recommendations couldn't be simpler. If you avoid sugar and junk food and follow the Honey Diet, you will lose weight – as much as 3 pounds (1.35kg) a week or a stone (6.35kg) a month. You will sleep like a baby, burning body fat throughout the night. And as an incredible bonus, you will be happier and far, far healthier because your brain isn't hungry. This means your stress levels will drop, and you will be doing the best you possibly can to protect yourself against degenerative diseases like diabetes, heart disease and Alzheimer's.

Try it. Make that switch from sugar to honey right now. The first thing you'll notice is the food cravings that might have been ruling your life will stop. You'll regain control over your eating, possibly for the first time in years.

You should start to lose weight immediately. You will certainly be sleeping better than you have since you were a child, happy in the knowledge that at night your body is operating exactly as it should – busying itself with recovery and repair and efficiently burning fat throughout the night as it does so.

As a bonus, you will also be reaping the multiple known health benefits of honey.

HONEY'S UNEXPECTED QUALITIES

1. Honey can protect the heart (studies show it has potent anti-adrenaline benefits)
2. Honey can lower blood pressure
3. Honey can reduce blood glucose levels
4. Honey is an antioxidant
5. Honey eases insomnia
6. Honey protects the brain (because it keeps the brain's feeder cells well stocked with fuel)
7. Honey can improve weight control
8. Honey improves memory and learning (because it supports brain function)
9. Honey protects the gut (it inhibits the growth of the bacterium called *Helicobacter pylori*, which is thought to trigger gastric ulcers)

10. Honey protects the liver
11. Honey is antibacterial (Manuka honey has been used in hospitals against MRSA infection)
12. Honey is antiviral
13. Honey is antifungal
14. Honey is anti-inflammatory
15. Honey may have anti-tumour effects

For every day and night you stick to the Honey Diet you can be confident that your body is NOT pumping out destructive stress hormones, your arteries are NOT furring up and your brain is NOT shrinking. By avoiding sugar and taking honey before bed each night, your memory will improve, you will feel brighter, more alert, and your body's ability to fight disease will get better and better every single day.

In the following chapters, I will show you exactly how the process works.

In chapter 1, I explain why, despite all your best intentions, a low-fat diet will never work and why sugar cravings are so infuriatingly difficult to ignore. I reveal how we have all been duped into believing that we should be filling up on bread, pasta and potatoes when these supposedly 'healthy' foods are, in fact, making us fat.

In chapter 2, I give you the secret of a good night's sleep, every night, for the rest of your life. And as a blissful bonus, I explain exactly how you can burn more body fat while you lie in bed, doing absolutely nothing, than you would pounding the pavements on a 10k run.

Chapter 3 is all about the miraculous powers of honey and the health benefits it brings. It really is so totally different from any other form of sugar, and I explain why, and how to use it for maximum effectiveness.

If you have already read enough and you are itching to get started RIGHT NOW on the Honey Diet, turn to chapter 4. Stock up on a large jar of honey, follow my guidelines, and tonight you could be sleeping like a baby, and wake tomorrow slimmer, healthier and efficiently fighting disease.

Chapter 5 is packed with practical tips for how to make the Honey Diet work for you.

Chapter 6 has ideas and inspiration for using honey in your everyday cooking.

Chapter 7 shows how the Honey Diet will boost your thinking, your powers of concentration, your memory, and could even reduce your risk of dementia and Alzheimer's.

Chapter 8 is all about a great big bonus of the honey diet – the fact that it really works hard to protect you against disease and ageing. Every day that you stick to the diet is a day when your body doesn't have to deal with the chemical cascade of stress hormones wreaking havoc on every tissue in your body. Over time, this lightening of the stress load will reduce your risk of degenerative diseases and slow the inevitable passage of time.

With honey on your side, you will lose weight (specifically body fat), you will sleep better, your body will become super-efficient at recovery and repair, and your brain will become sharper, faster and more focussed. It is quite a bonus for such a small lifestyle change!

A slender, healthy future is in your hands and the Honey Diet holds the key.

Chapter I

THE KEY TO WEIGHT LOSS

Wouldn't it be wonderful if our bodies worked as they should? We'd feel so healthy, we'd sleep so peacefully. We would be able to eat whenever we felt hungry, but never gain weight. And we wouldn't have to worry about life-threatening obesity-related disorders such as diabetes, heart disease or Alzheimer's.

But there's no getting away from the fact that we have all started to expand alarmingly in size.

When I was a schoolboy in the 1950s, there was usually one overweight child in every class, most often a boy – a kind of Billy Bunter figure. But since the mid-1970s, almost everyone seems to have expanded and I've noticed a rapid and steady increase in the size of the people around me.

Primary public health concerns always used to focus on conditions like bronchitis, smoking, heart disease, colds and flu, childhood vaccinations and the avoidance of major diseases such as polio and TB. When I was a young pharmacist in the 1960s, we mostly sold painkillers, cough mixtures, antacids and laxatives. But in the 1970s, that began to change. From 1975 onwards, weight control became a leading topic of public and media attention. The word 'diet' entered the vocabulary and new diets became an almost daily media focus. We were selling saccharin tablets and issuing prescriptions for appetite-suppressing amphetamines. By the 1980s, Slimfast had arrived from the USA and was taking the country by storm.

But still waistlines continued to expand.

Diabetes went from being a rare metabolic condition, to something extremely common – even among young children. Then, more slowly, but just as ominously, a new word entered our vocabulary – Alzheimer's. We knew about dementia, but it wasn't something we worried about. But by the end of the twentieth century, Alzheimer's was everywhere. We all knew of someone who was living with a hideously gradual deterioration of their mind and many of us (rightly so) feared for the long-term future of our own sanity.

Millions of pounds of public funds are continually being pumped into devising a coherent public health message that could bring us back from the bad-health brink, and avert what looks like an impending obesity epidemic.

The message has always been simple: you can avoid being fat by balancing calories in and calories out. The problem, the authorities persistently say, is human fallibility. We're all too greedy and lazy. We eat too much and we exercise too little.

Over the last few decades, millions of us have heeded the Government's advice, pulling out our trainers and jogging to work, or signing up at a shiny new health club and sweating our way through interminable exercise classes.

We have also become obsessed with diets and a whole new diet-food industry has evolved, with big food manufacturers cashing in on our national obsession with cutting fat and calories.

Diets and diet foods have become a massive multi-million-pound international business. Slimming books regularly and consistently top the bestseller lists and so desperate is the public quest for the diet holy grail – effortless weight loss – that the circulation figures of national newspapers can be significantly boosted by a tasty diet serialization.

But despite this gargantuan investment, nothing seems to be working and we are STILL getting fatter. The latest UK figures show that 65 per cent of men and 58 per cent of women are now classed as overweight or obese, and the figures continue to rise.

So what on earth has been happening? Where have we been going so very, very wrong?

FAT IS BAD – OR IS IT?

There is no doubt that being overweight puts you at risk of a plethora of potentially fatal illnesses. But specialists still can't agree on which aspect of the way we eat is causing us to gain weight, and triggering disease.

The link between diet and heart disease dates back to the 1950s when saturated fat came under the spotlight as the big dietary evil. This type of fat, found in meat and dairy products, was believed to directly increase levels of heart-clogging cholesterol in the blood.

A scientist called Dr Norman Jolliffe came up with a theory that Americans were getting fat and becoming increasingly prone to heart disease because they ate too many high-fat hamburgers. He worked with the New York Health Department to devise a low-fat diet he called 'the Prudent Diet'.

Dr Jolliffe set up a long-term study whereby he fed one group of businessmen a low-fat diet (margarine instead of butter, breakfast cereal instead of eggs, and fish instead of beef) and another group stayed on a 'normal' higher fat diet (meat three times a day). After 5 years, the men on the lower fat diet DID show improved cholesterol levels, which was (and to a large extent still is) believed to be a good thing because it was thought to indicate that they had a lower risk of heart disease.

However, 8 men (out of 814) on the low-fat diet actually DIED of heart disease during the study, whereas none of the men on the high-fat diet died. Dr Jolliffe couldn't explain this and the New York Health Department focussed instead on the small reduction in cholesterol their diet had produced. They concluded, irrefutably, that a low-fat diet was a really useful means of reducing heart disease risk and weight.

This thinking still feeds into the 'fat is bad for you' debate today.

In 1972, a British scientist called John Yudkin wrote a ground-breaking book called *Pure, White and Deadly*, which argued that refined sugar, and NOT fat, was the decisive factor in trig-gering heart disease. This was highly contentious stuff.

Meanwhile, a famous American physiologist, Ancel Keys (who was at that time a bit of a dietetics hero for his sterling work in nutrition and starvation during WW2), set out his stall in opposition to Yudkin, perpetuating the old 'fat is bad' theory.

Keys' seminal *Seven Countries Study*, published in the 1980s, demonized fat – particularly saturated fat – by highlighting those nations where a high intake of dietary fats was linked to high levels of heart disease. It was compelling evidence but, increas-ingly, scientists have questioned the validity of his findings. It turns out Keys' study excluded results from certain countries where high-fat diets (such as those of Inuits – natives of the most northern regions of North America, Canada, Greenland

and Russia – whose diets are up to 75 per cent fat) did not create a heart attack epidemic.

Also, Keys' research did not consider the separate impact of sugar on the nations he studied.

The authorities of the time, backed by a multi-million-dollar food industry that had a significant interest in encouraging us to continue consuming sugar in large quantities, decided to favour Keys' fat theory over Yudkin's sugar theory, and Yudkin's work was marginalized and discredited.

Having invested their reputations in their fat theory, the denizens of the scientific establishment rubbished the views of anyone who dared to oppose it, and did everything they could to discredit them.

By the 1980s, LOW FAT was the key health message and the big obesity-busting drive worldwide.

The 'ideal' diet, we were told (and are still being told), is low in fat. We should, they say, be filling up on carbohydrates. The food industry helpfully altered its recipes. Fats were removed from all sorts of processed foods and, in an effort to make low-fat food edible, sugar was added to almost everything (both sweet and savoury).

Now, after decades of low-fat, high-sugar consumption, our tastes and eating habits have gradually changed. We have become carbohydrate-driven. Wherever you are in the world, there's a strong chance you'll eat a carbohydrate-heavy breakfast (cereal, toast, muffins), lunch (sandwiches) and dinner (chips, pasta, rice) and snack on volumes of white flour and sugar (biscuits, cakes, pastries, sweets) in-between. You'll find fast-food outlets in every city and growing populations worldwide inadvertently hooked on easy-to-eat high-sugar foods.

Americans now consume 40kg of added sugars a year and we Brits are little better, getting through a shocking 29kg –

some 4½ stone – of the white stuff every year. Even China, which you'd think had enough of a cultural heritage to steer around the surge towards processed food, looks set to become the world's largest consumer of sugar by 2020. Its demand doubles every 20 years, and all the predictions are that personal consumption will rapidly exceed that of the West.

But obesity figures continue to rise, and heart disease remains the number one killer.

It is quite clear that something is going wrong.

Could it be that, through relentless advertising and ubiquitous availability – not to mention funding and support of government bodies and the scientific community – the food industry is steering us in the wrong direction?

THE KETONE COPS: A PLOT AGAINST ATKINS

Dr Robert Atkins was, in my opinion, a man ahead of his time. In the 1970s, the US cardiologist suspected the low-fat diet message might not be right, and devised his now famous Atkins Diet.

His solution to the obesity crisis was to create a diet that dramatically reduced carbohydrates (cutting out potatoes, bread, pasta, rice and even starchy vegetables like carrots and sweet corn) and replaced them with fats (even saturated fat) and large quantities of protein (meat, fish etc).

It was shocking, and counterintuitive, but his diet worked. Millions followed it and many lost significant amounts of weight. They found it easy, and were very happy.

Dr Atkins was even able to show that the high-fat diet did NOT increase heart disease risk.

That's a good thing, right?

Apparently not. The medical and scientific establishments were outraged and many pilloried Atkins.

I was a practising pharmacist at the height of the Atkins phenomenon and quizzed countless professionals about the regime. Without exception, they condemned it as dangerous. If further pressed to explain, the universal response was, 'Too much protein is bad for you.'

After a few years, the Atkins regime fell out of favour, to the point that when Robert Atkins died (of brain trauma following a fall) his company eventually sued for bankruptcy. What went wrong?

Recent science shows that the Atkins Diet faded from public support for one very simple reason: a no-carbohydrate diet is almost impossible to sustain for any length of time.

The problem is we really do need SOME carbohydrates in our diet. Not only is it very difficult to survive in a modern world without carbohydrates (or at least, resist their relentlessly ubiquitous availability), but man did not evolve to eat like this long term.

However, there is plenty of evidence to suggest that Atkins was on the right track (**see notes page 126**), and I have incorporated some elements of his thinking into the Honey Diet. The Honey Diet is not an Atkins-type diet – I definitely do not advocate banning carbohydrates – but it works by *reducing* the intake of sugar and refined carbohydrates, which, I am absolutely convinced, are the driving force of modern weight gain.

SUGAR – THE TRUE EVIL

For most of our evolutionary history, sugars and carbohydrate foods have been in short supply. We may have foraged for fruits and berries, but we had no access to the high-energy grains and rice that have been introduced relatively recently into the human diet.

After WW2, sugar became available to everyone in increasing amounts, prices came right down and new processed foods were created to tempt us. Gradually the consumption of sugars rose.

The UK Government-recommended food pyramid has carbohydrates at the base, therefore advocating that bread, pasta, rice and potatoes should form the bulk of our food intake.

But whenever we eat refined breads, pasta, rice, sweets, dried fruits, biscuits, cakes, pies, spreads, jams, cereals and other high-calorie foods and snacks, the sugar levels in our blood escalate. The body responds by pumping out the hormone insulin, which very cleverly clears the sugar out of the blood and stores it as fat.

The problem is that we have been misled by 50 years of poor nutritional advice into believing that carbohydrate foods are good for us. We get fat not just from too much fat in food, but from sugar in the diet that the body converts to fat.

GLUTTONY AND GREED?

It is a very common misconception that if you get fat, you must be greedy. But I really don't believe humans are greedy. Unlike most animals, we share food with family, friends and others on a daily basis, and especially on festive occasions.

Yet suddenly we are eating far more food than we need – what's going on?

Clearly, one reason we over-consume is because, unlike previous generations, we have unlimited access to low-cost, high-calorie food. Snacks can be bought at every filling station and 24-hour corner shop. At any moment, day or night, we are never more than a few metres from a readily accessible source of high-sugar food. Gone are the days of three solid home-cooked meals a day eaten at the kitchen table such as existed when I was a boy. Now we eat all day long.

US anti-sugar campaigner Professor Robert Lustig blames what he calls 'Big Food' – the major global producers of processed, high-sugar, high-fat food, which, he says, are no better than tobacco manufacturers, pumping out unhealthy, addictive products at a hefty profit, unwilling to change.

He's right. Yes, we are consuming more food than at any time in our history. But I believe the problem is not greediness, it is hunger. Not body hunger (we eat far too much for many of us to even remember what that feels like), but BRAIN hunger.

WHY OUR BRAINS ARE HUNGRY

I have spent the last 15 years studying diet and metabolism and I am convinced that the problem – for everyone – lies in the way our bodies react to the sugar overload of the modern diet.

In the 1950s an eminent American nutritionist called Jean Mayer developed an interesting new theory of appetite control. He worked out that the brain (not the stomach) was involved in stimulating and quelling appetite, and that the level of glucose in the blood that reached the brain played an important role in the process.

He believed that when we haven't eaten for a while, and levels of blood glucose fall, the brain (which needs a steady stream of glucose as fuel and is hypersensitive to even a tiny drop in supply) detects this drop. It sets in motion a chain of commands in the form of stress and appetite hormones, which trigger all the requirements for food seeking and food consumption – foraging and hunting (or, in modern-day language, impossible to resist cravings).

It is no coincidence that when cravings strike, they will most likely be for something sugary – very often chocolate. The brain is under no illusion that it needs sugar and it needs it fast. The problem is we don't stop at one biscuit or one piece of chocolate. When cravings strike, we very often eat far, far too much.

My research shows that when we eat quantities of high-sugar food, the body is flooded with excess glucose. If this got to the brain, it would overload it, damaging delicate tissues. So, instead, the brain triggers an extremely clever defence mechanism.

THE iPUMP

As I suggested earlier, in a healthy person eating a healthy diet, there is an efficient transport mechanism called the 'cerebral glucose pump' (I call it the iPump), which acts as a sensor, ensuring meticulously measured amounts of glucose flow from the blood to the neurones – the workhorse cells of the brain. But a great surge of glucose in the blood will flick a switch and suppress the iPump.

The iPump is, in fact, made up of millions and millions of microscopic pumps in certain cells of the brain called glial cells. These are the 'feeder cells' of the brain, which outnumber the 'thinking cells' (the neurones) by as many as ten to one. Their only job is to minutely control the fuel supply to the neurones, so the brain works as it should.

THE iPUMP IN ACTION

In the brain neurones do the thinking, and glial cells protect and feed them. Each glial cell contains a microscopic iPump which monitors sugar levels in the blood, and feeds fuel to the neurones. If the iPump detects too much sugar and insulin, it shuts down to protect the neurone from overload, and allows only emergency fuel rations through.

Neurones: the work horses of the brain

Glial cells: feeder cells for the neurones

HIGH-SUGAR DIET
EXCESS GLUCOSE/INSULIN

HONEY DIET
NORMAL GLUCOSE/INSULIN

iPump OFF

ON iPump

GLIAL CELL

GLIAL CELL

Brain fuel

Brain fuel

Stressed Hungry Neurone

Happy Healthy Neurone

© SCOOP EDITORIAL & DESIGN LTD.

Any energy-using system, whether electrical or mechanical, has to control its energy source. If the flow is too high or strong, a fail-safe device will normally be triggered to prevent disaster.

It's the same in the brain. A sugar overload will trip the switch on the iPump, blocking all but the merest trickle of fuel to the brain.

Once the iPump is suppressed, the brain's fuel supply is reduced to the bare minimum it needs to function (like the dim battery-powered emergency light that stays on after a power-cut), effectively cutting off access to this excessive flood of blood glucose.

This means that no matter how much food you now eat, your brain will be kept stable, and protected from harmful excess. It is a great bit of self-preservation for the brain, and it makes perfect, logical sense.

The brain clearly evolved this system in a time when food was pretty scarce. It solves the problem of potential overload because the iPump will remain shut off for as long as the eating of high-sugar foods continues. For centuries, this food glut would not last long and food would only be plentiful for a short time (after a hunt or, in more recent times, a harvest). The food would then run out and blood sugar levels would drop. The iPump would kick back into action, the neurones would be fed once more, and everything would be back to normal.

I think this has only become a problem now because our brain's delicate system simply can't cope with the vast quantity of food we eat today.

If you find yourself standing in front of a huge buffet table groaning with food, or in a shopping centre where every other outlet is selling sweet, fatty, easily accessible deliciousness, most of us will just continue eating. But do what your body is telling you and keep on returning to that buffet table, over and over again, and your iPump will stay tripped, protecting the brain from this on-going sugar glut. This means that only the tiniest trickle of fuel can get through to the brain – just enough for it to function in 'emergency mode'.

If the iPump stays tripped, it won't be long before the brain becomes hungry, as the starved neurones inevitably send out emergency signals to try to boost their fuel supply once more. Which is why that buffet or those doughnuts always seem so tempting.

The brain is extremely selfish and thinks only of its own survival at the expense of the rest of the body. A hungry brain will set up a stress response to encourage you to eat more food, triggering the release of appetite hormones.

But each new episode of eating only increases the power load, short-circuiting the brain and making us hungrier. This can lead to a vicious cycle of uncontrolled eating while the iPump remains permanently suppressed. I believe it is this that explains the now worryingly common phenomenon of human giants who are too big for normal domestic life, bedridden and managed by mechanical cranes, who never, ever stop eating.

ARE CRAVINGS ALL IN THE MIND?

Nutritionists and health professionals talk about cravings as 'psychological hunger' and for decades we have bemoaned our weak willpower and ridiculous inability to resist the chocolate bar or burger or large bag of popcorn that we really don't need.

But the urge continually to eat is not an imagined hunger. We really can feel properly hungry, even after gorging ourselves at a big meal.

If you eat an unhealthy, high-sugar diet, there is every chance that your brain will be enduring a slow state of gradual starvation. You will have triggered your iPump to switch off and your body may be awash with glucose, but your brain will always be hungry.

When scientists use brain scans to investigate what happens when people are shown images of hamburgers, cakes and biscuits, they find that different areas of the brain light up for those prone to obesity.

A 2013 study at the University of Colorado showed groups of overweight and slim people images of high-calorie foods both before and after they had eaten a meal. The brain scans of the overweight people revealed a stronger response in the reward areas of their brain than it did with the slim people.

It seems that if you are overweight, your iPump is likely to be on permanent switch-off, your brain chronically hungry, and therefore much more focussed on food.

Certainly you'd expect the brain to show a greater response to food BEFORE a meal, but incredibly, in overweight people, the same heightened response showed AFTER the meal, too. It is clear that something is going fundamentally wrong.

Interestingly, it is SUGARY foods that trigger the most heightened response in overweight people – just the fuel supply the brain is urging you to choose.

Cravings are clearly a physiological, not merely a psychological, phenomenon.

When you walk into a burger bar, for instance, you will probably be enjoying the thought of your favourite cheeseburger. The closer you get to the food, the more relaxed you might feel. This is because the anticipation will have kicked off a cascade of hormones, such as serotonin, the feel-good hormone, that improves mood and prepares your body for taking in the food.

In your brain you will also have activated the dopamine reward system, a hormone sequence that causes us to seek more of the same (dopamine is a key hormone in many forms of addiction).

So dopamine floods the brain's receptors and makes the brain relaxed and happy – it knows the energy supply that it needs is about to be replenished. At this moment, just before your favourite meal arrives, you will rarely feel better.

Then, before you peel off the wrappers, your pancreas will secrete a tide of the hormone insulin in anticipation of the sugars it is about to receive. Ten minutes later, when you have finished eating, you will feel momentarily satisfied, but keep an eye on your watch. Fifteen minutes on, you might begin to feel different – perhaps slightly anxious.

The flood of processed food will have hiked your blood sugar and therefore insulin levels and, in all likelihood, your iPump will have switched off to protect your brain from a potential sugar overload. But now your brain isn't happy. Because of the iPump, it didn't receive the sugar boost it was expecting, and now it wants to send you back for another try.

Clearly something has gone wrong. Your blood is coursing with extra glucose and fats so there's no shortage of energy, but you've tripped your iPump switch and your brain – the greediest organ in the body by a very long way – is still hungry.

THE HUNGRY BRAIN IN ACTION

During the Edinburgh Festival of 2011, I met some friends in a cafe that was part of a theatre complex. Next to our group I spotted a number of young actors discussing their play and preparing to rehearse in a theatre next door. Among the group was a young woman in her mid-twenties, who was clearly overweight but who ate continuously throughout their discussion. When the group entered the theatre to rehearse their play, she popped back out, opened her bag and removed some bread, then spread it with butter and toppings and consumed the makeshift sandwich rapidly (in a few seconds) before going back into the theatre. Fifteen minutes later, the episode was repeated, and again every 15 minutes for 2 hours.

This, to me, was the iPump in action. I believe that every time she popped out for a snack, the energy from the food she ate was not reaching her brain in sufficient quantities to tell it to switch off the hunger signals.

In fact, each new round of sandwiches was simply adding to her appetite. Her sugary fillings and the white pappy bread were giving a swift hike in blood glucose, which was suppressing her iPump and inhibiting sugar supply to her brain. She was already overweight, so very likely to be suffering from insulin resistance (most overweight people are), a condition that makes iPump suppression even more likely.

Her brain was probably starving and sending out impossible to resist cravings, with each new round of eating adding to the problem, and promoting repeated episodes of even more eating.

It is quite clear that the woman's refuelling systems were on full alert, forcing her to eat more and more food, but the message obviously wasn't getting to her brain.

Chapter 2

SLEEP LIKE A BABY

Most of us think of sleep as a time of rest for the body and brain, but, in fact, nothing could be further from the truth. We might be unconscious, but at night we couldn't be busier. Cells have to be cleared of damaged tissue and toxins, and cells, muscles, even tiny sinews, have to be repaired. The process of night-time recovery is a huge logistical and energy-demanding enterprise of demolition, transportation and rebuilding, so the brain remains extremely active throughout, conducting the whole process to ensure we wake up in the morning in tiptop mental and physical condition and ready to face the day.

If everything is working properly, this essential process uses body fat as fuel. So, on a good night, you should be burning considerable quantities of body fat while you are lying flat on your back in bed.

It is an amazing bonus if you want to lose weight, and one that I believe many of us could be missing out on. Because, if you really want to lose weight, changing your diet and adding exercise are rarely sufficient – you need to be getting 8 hours of quality sleep every night if you are going to take full advantage of this fantastic nocturnal fat-burning opportunity.

HOW YOUR BODY CAN BURN MORE FAT SLEEPING THAN EXERCISING

In a BBC *Horizon* programme, medical journalist Dr Michael Mosley conducted an experiment with specialists at Glasgow University that showed that a tough 90-minute workout only burned 9.5g of body fat. This was a disappointingly small amount considering his hour and a half of sweaty effort. But, fascinatingly, when the scientists measured Dr Mosley's metabolism as he slept that night, they found he burned five times as much body fat (49g).

An hour and a half of exercise is a lot by anyone's standards, but other studies confirm Mosley's findings, showing that even if you haven't exercised AT ALL during the day, you could still be burning considerable quantities of body fat during the night.

The studies vary, but I think it is possible to burn around 65g of body fat during the night. That's seven times the fat-burning potential of a 90-minute workout – and you will have to impart exactly ZERO effort to do it! In one week, you could burn 455g (that's 1lb) of fat and in a month you could shift 3kg of pure fat (½ stone), without dieting or exercising at all.

It sounds too good to be true and, yes, there is a caveat that is crucial to the Honey Diet. For proper night-time fat burning to happen like this, your body has to be in perfect balance with NO chance that your brain could be allowed to get hungry during the night.

This is because if you sleep badly, or fitfully, if you go to bed hungry, or if your brain starts to feel hungry or stressed during the night, the resulting stress hormones immediately halt any repair and recovery process so that fat burning just won't happen. Studies show that fat loss will occur only during slow-wave sleep, which is when the body's recovery and repair process really gets into gear. This deep sleep doesn't happen if you are lying down with your eyes closed (pretending to sleep) or if you sleep poorly.

I am convinced that one of the reasons we are all gaining weight so frighteningly fast is because so many of us are losing the ability to sleep soundly and well. Repair and recovery aren't happening as they should, and we're not burning fat at night.

THE LETHAL EFFECT OF POOR SLEEP ON OUR BODIES

Aside from missing out on the fat-burning bonus, poor sleep is catastrophic for our mental and physical health.

There is no doubt that sleep deprivation is very, very bad for the brain. It affects memory, learning, our ability to concentrate, to understand, our reaction times, and even our ability to perform perfectly ordinary daily tasks. Any new parent knows you only have to endure a few broken nights before you start feeling fatigued, confused, disorientated, sometimes nauseous, and your brain just seems to stop wanting to work properly.

It is no wonder sleep deprivation is used as an instrument of torture.

But only in the last decade have scientists pondered the possibility that poor sleep might ALSO have strong links with diseases such as obesity, diabetes and heart disease. And this may be only the tip of a disease-iceberg that includes osteoporosis, depression, infertility, poor immune function, compromised memory and cognition and neurodegenerative diseases like Alzheimer's.

Studies have also shown that sleep deprivation prevents the formation of new brain cells, vital to new learning and memory consolidation. This is because when we sleep, our short-term memory should be transferred from the holding bay in the brain (the hippocampus) to the cortex, where it becomes long-term memory. With poor quality sleep, this process can't happen properly.

Chronic sleep deprivation is having a silent, but lethal effect on our bodies and brains. It is certainly clear to me that we'd all be a lot healthier, would live longer, we'd age more slowly and gain less weight if only we got enough sleep.

WHY POOR SLEEP MAKES US FAT

Numerous studies have linked poor sleep with weight gain. For instance, in 2008 scientists from Cleveland University in Ohio looked at thirty-six studies from around the world and concluded, 'Short sleep duration appears independently associated with weight gain, particularly in younger age groups.'

If we've slept badly, we tend to eat more the next day. We might think we're just trying to give ourselves a sugar boost, but I'm convinced we are not consciously driving the process – our stressed and hungry brain is.

A Chicago University academic, Eve Van Cauter, conducted an experiment where she took otherwise healthy young men and interrupted their sleep patterns for only two nights. She found that sleep deprivation raised levels of the appetite hormone ghrelin and the poor sleep-deprived students reported increased levels of hunger (up by 24 per cent) and appetite (23 per cent), and strong cravings for calorie-dense food (from 33 to 45 per cent).

The implications are clear and worrying. If this is the result of only two nights of sleep restriction, what can we expect from the chronic sleep loss that most of us endure? You just have to look at the number of overweight people around you to see the results.

WHY CAN'T WE SLEEP?

Sadly, it seems a good night's sleep is increasingly becoming a rare and precious thing and few of us in the West ever get the full 8 hours of recovery and repair we should.

According to the Great British Sleep Survey (of 2011) more than half of British adults are unable to secure a good night's sleep, with women being three times more vulnerable than men. Twenty-five per cent of those who reported insomnia problems confessed they had been living with sleep deprivation for more than a decade.

In the USA a similar crisis is emerging. According to the American Sleep Association, most Americans fall short on sleep by 2 hours each night.

We might blame an active lifestyle, too much rich food, an overstimulated brain, the menopause, the light, noise, traffic or birds for keeping us awake at night, but I am convinced that our modern epidemic of insomnia is much more often caused by one (or both) of two factors:

1. Our modern high-carbohydrate, junk food diet, which trips the iPump at night, triggering a dramatic cascade of hormonal and chemical events that makes us sleep fitfully.
2. Eating our last meal of the day in the early evening, meaning there are insufficient fuel reserves to feed the brain properly throughout the night, triggering a dramatic cascade of hormonal and chemical events that makes us sleep fitfully.

THE iPUMP AT NIGHT

If you've got into the habit of eating processed, high-sugar junk food and washing your evening meal down with a glass or two of wine, there's a strong chance the flood of blood sugar will have tripped your iPump.

This means you might drop off to sleep quite happily, but yours will not necessarily be a sound or restful sleep. With your iPump switched off, your brain will be receiving the merest trickle of fuel, and will very soon become hungry.

It will trigger the release of stress hormones to try to call up glucose reserves from the liver, but when your iPump is switched off, even these supplies won't get through. Your brain gets hungrier still. Stress hormones will be sent out with instructions to break down muscle protein into fuel, but that glucose won't get through the iPump barrier either.

You will most likely spend the night sleeping fitfully with stress hormones washing around your system wreaking havoc, and wake up feeling nauseated, groggy and hungry.

This is the fastest possible route to weight gain.

If you eat well, but early in the evening (as health experts have long advised), you could fall foul of a similar chemical cascade because your brain is likely to suspect that there isn't enough fuel in its reserve tanks to keep it going until breakfast.

THE GREEDY BRAIN

The human brain may be small, but this bundle of cells is so complex that it burns up twenty-two times the energy of any cell in any other tissue in the body. And if it is hungry, it will be very, very demanding.

Although it makes up only 2 per cent of our total body mass (weighing about 1.5kg), the average human brain consumes approximately 6g of glucose per hour – equivalent to 24 calories. So over a 24-hour period, the brain will typic-ally demand 576 calories of glucose merely to function and survive. This is equivalent to 384 calories for each kg of brain.

If the rest of our body demanded fuel at that rate, it would mean that an 11¾ stone (75kg) man would need to consume 28,000 calories every day (twenty-eight loaves of bread).

Because of these massive fuel demands, the human brain exists in an exquisitely fine balance. It MUST have a steady supply of glucose to keep it functioning properly – not too much and not too little.

Get the balance exactly right and the brain can get on with its job of controlling everything you say, think and do, masterminding the action of every single cell, nerve, hormone, reaction and sinew in the body. At night, its most important job is to orchestrate the repair and recovery process around the body – the process that burns body fat.

Unfortunately, it is very easy to get the balance wrong.

The brain is incredibly delicate and sensitive, prone to huge overreactions if it suspects there's a shortage of fuel.

It only has very small energy reserves – enough for about 8 to 10 minutes' thinking time. If its delicate sensors pick up the possibility that stocks are starting to get a little low (if we haven't eaten for a few hours), it will react swiftly and dramatically to try to rectify the situation and safeguard the perfectly regulated supply of fuel it needs.

It sends out stress hormones with instructions to call up reserve supplies of glucose held in special glycogen stores in the liver.

But the liver's glycogen stores are not very large, and they are often plundered by other parts of the body, such as muscles, heart and kidneys, as a reserve energy supply.

At maximum capacity, the glycogen stores can hold around 50 to 75g of glucose, but at night, when you're not eating (and thereby continually replenishing them), the stores can deplete at a rate of 10g per hour.

For fat burning to happen effectively at night, the brain must be happy, and this means it must be well stocked with enough fuel to keep it ticking along nicely for the full 8 hours until breakfast.

WHAT TIME'S DINNER?

When you eat your evening meal, the glucose in your blood will be directed straight to the liver to stock up your glycogen stores ready for the night fast. But if you are in the habit of eating at 5 or 6pm (as health experts recommend), there simply won't be enough reserves in the liver to supply the brain throughout the whole night.

For decades, health gurus have been advising us to eat 'breakfast like a king, lunch like a prince and dinner like a pauper', to make sure we avoid a carbohydrate-heavy evening meal that would just turn to fat overnight.

But I believe this advice has been adding to our obesity problem, and the old custom in some parts of the world of eating a main meal late at night has health benefits that we haven't fully appreciated.

For thousands of years, people living in Spain, Italy and southern France would wait until 10 or 11pm to sit down for dinner. This meant it was perfectly normal for generations to efficiently restock their liver and recharge their brain's energy stores before they went to bed. Without them realising it, this would ensure the brain was supplied with a steady and controlled source of energy throughout the night, allowing for quality sleep, efficient processing and perfect balance.

However, over the last 50 years, the people of the southern Mediterranean have begun to abandon the tradition of a late supper. Combine this with the increasingly widespread popularity of junk food, and you can see why the southern Mediterranean has become the fastest-growing region in Europe for weight gain, diabetes and dementias (Spain, for instance, now has the third highest incidence of childhood obesity in the world and looks set to overtake even America).

DON'T SHUN CARBOHYDRATES IN THE EVENING

Studies now show that eating *some* carbohydrates with your evening meal is the best way to stock up the liver's glycogen stores for the night. This ensures a steady trickle of fuel to the brain, no need for the nocturnal stress response and efficient activation of the whole recovery and repair process (which – bonus! – burns fat as fuel).

One notable study took two groups of obese policemen and put them on calorie-controlled diets. The control group were allowed to spread their carbohydrate consumption throughout the day, but the test group could only eat their carbs for dinner (with the expectation that they would find it the most difficult to lose weight). The results after 6 months confounded conventional wisdom. The late-night carb eaters showed greater weight loss, but they also showed metabolic changes beneficial to their health.

The authors stated: 'A simple dietary manipulation of carbohydrate distribution appears to have additional benefits when compared to a conventional weight-loss diet in individuals suffering from obesity.'

BRING BACK THE SIESTA

The fabulous southern Mediterranean tradition of an afternoon siesta has rapidly fallen out of favour. These days, most people who do take a break after lunch would rather watch television or fiddle around with Facebook than have a snooze. And studies show that this means they could be missing out on the health benefits of an afternoon nap.

Studies show that actually sleeping during a short siesta burns as much as three times the body fat of 'resting awake' (dozing, reading or watching television). This, I believe, is because a proper sleep means the brain is allowed to get on with what it is supposed to do (the recovery process that burns body fat).

A large Greek study found that a post-lunch siesta created a 37 per cent reduction in the risk of heart disease. I am convinced that this is because sleep allows the body to work effectively and resting properly gives the body a break from the adrenal stress hormones, which are major contributors to heart disease.

After a healthy midday meal, the liver's glycogen stores will be stocked, which means the brain has an assured supply of fuel and will be in exactly the right state to start instructing recovery and repair. That familiar feeling of torpor and drowsiness that invades us in the after-lunch hours is simply the brain signalling that it is fuelled and relaxed – an excellent time for a snatched bit of recovery, repair and fat burning.

WHY HONEY HELPS YOU BURN BODY FAT AT NIGHT

It is an incredible untapped weight-loss bonus that a good night's sleep uses body fat to fuel the nightly repair and recovery process. But studies (which date back as far as the 1950s) confirm that this will only happen effectively if the glycogen stores in the liver are full-to-bursting before you go to bed.

This is because the glycogen stores are absolutely essential reserve energy tanks for the brain. The brain will not allow repair and recovery (and therefore fat burning) to happen if it is hungry. The second it suspects its fuel supply might be compromised, it will set off chemical reactions to get fuel from other sources and will, every time, abort recovery in the process.

If the brain's sensors pick up the fact that the glycogen stores are getting low, it will go into overdrive, calling on glucose from any other available source.

Reaching for bigger guns, the brain's next step is to call up the stress hormone cortisol (which works in combination with glucagon) to start to manufacture new glucose by breaking down muscle fibres elsewhere in the body (it's a kind of self-cannibalism).

All the time they are flooding the system, these stress hormones will be disrupting your sleep, damaging delicate tissues throughout your body and – significantly – they will be stopping the repair and recovery process happening, which means you WON'T be burning fat.

You can very effectively fill your liver glycogen tanks before you go to bed by EITHER eating a nutritious and balanced LATE evening meal (the body directs glucose from your food into the glycogen stores) or 'cheating' by taking a few spoons of honey before you go to sleep.

Unlike the sugar in a sugary night-time drink, most of the glucose in honey goes directly to the glycogen stores of the liver – just where it is needed as the brain's reserve night-time fuel supply.

This ensures that the brain has the fuel it needs, the iPump will work efficiently and effectively, and the fat-burning recovery process will occur as it should.

I've calculated that the perfect amount of honey you need to restock the liver's glycogen stores is 1 to 2 tablespoons (50g) of honey before you go to bed. This is exactly enough to activate perfect sleep and the recovery process, which means you are likely to wake the following morning bright, alert, mentally focussed and, after a Honey Diet breakfast, confident, balanced and ready to face the day.

On the occasions when you do have a nourishing late evening meal, you may not need to restock your glycogen stores with honey. However, a teaspoon or two of honey in hot water WILL send you off to sleep perfectly.

> ## CASE STUDY
>
> Rachel, 26, dropped more than half a stone (3.5kg) from over
> 13 stone (85kg) to 12¾ stone (81.5kg) and shrank
> 3cm off her hips and 4cm off her waist in 2 weeks.
>
> *'I've been reducing my carbohydrate intake and loading up on
> vegetables instead, particularly in the evenings. I really enjoy
> the habit of honey at night and I am convinced that it ensures
> I sleep better (and I can't resist the temptation of the possibility
> that it might mean I burn more fat while I sleep).'*

WHY HONEY MAKES YOU DROWSY

In 1950, two researchers from Sheffield University and the University of Alexandria found that we burn more fat at night if the whole process is kick-started by a spike of glucose at bedtime.

When we eat a spoonful of honey or sip it stirred into a hot drink, the sweetness briefly provides the small glucose spike, which stimulates the release of insulin.

This is useful, because a little bit of insulin is needed for the body to trigger the release of the sleepy hormone, melatonin. Very helpfully, melatonin will then trigger the release of the growth hormones that kick off the incredibly beneficial recovery phase that burns body fat.

This is possibly why honey has been used for centuries (often in milk) as a late-night drink.

As a convenient side effect, these growth hormones then inhibit the production of insulin, thereby protecting the body from its ill effects and preventing the overloading of your delicate system with glucose and insulin.

MELATONIN, LIGHT POLLUTION . . . AND HONEY

There may be many things keeping you awake, but I believe 'light pollution' plays a part. One of the key reasons we don't sleep as well as we should (and don't burn fat like we should) is because we have drifted so far from the natural 'awake during daylight hours and asleep when it's dark' pattern of our ancestors.

With bright street lights everywhere and the lights of electronic gadgetry in every bedroom, we are rarely truly in the dark. Artificial light might give us the opportunity of extending our waking hours, but it reduces the time of proper darkness, and this puts us at risk of becoming increasingly disconnected from our natural environment and the vital regulation this provides.

The problem is that the sleep hormone, melatonin, needs darkness to function – its release is controlled by the light/dark cycle of day and night. The hormone is produced by the pineal gland in the brain, but only when the retina at the back of the eye detects low levels of light. When light strikes the retina, melatonin cannot be produced.

However, darkness is not enough. Melatonin is not produced if the brain is hungry. A spoonful of honey before bed is enough to give the brain the energy it needs to trigger the melatonin release that guarantees restful sleep. Is it any wonder then that milk with honey has long been regarded as a perfect bedtime drink?

That spoonful of honey is a worthy investment because melatonin doesn't just aid recovery – it improves the function of the iPump, it is a potent antioxidant and it improves immune function. It may even be a useful tool in the treatment of Alzheimer's.

If you really want to maximize the beneficial effects of melatonin, it's a good idea to get all electrical devices (computers, TVs etc) out of the bedroom. And don't think that a relaxing alcoholic drink before bed is going to help because studies show that alcohol suppresses melatonin production.

CASE STUDY

Chloe, 41, a PR executive from London, lost 9 pounds (4.1kg) on the Honey Diet in 8 weeks, but noticed the biggest change in her sleep patterns.

'Insomnia used to be a big problem for me,' she says. 'I'd typically drop off in front of the TV at about 9pm, then drag myself to bed at midnight, but wake at 4am and lie there worrying, frustrated and annoyed with myself. If I did doze off at dawn, I'd be woken by the alarm feeling awful. Since trying the Honey Diet all that has changed. Now I go to bed at around 10.30 with my honey drink and more often than not I sleep right through until 6 or 7am. It's amazing! I think honey is a natural, healthy food and it satisfies my sweet cravings. I don't feel I'm on a diet so I don't feel any need to stop.'

CAN'T SLEEP, WON'T SLEEP
(TREATING INSOMNIA)

I am convinced that taking 2 tablespoons of honey at night – every night – is a more effective cure for insomnia than any pill or potion. It is delicious, easy and has NO side effects!

Insomnia has always been a problem and since the nineteenth century it has been regarded by the medical professions as an issue that can be effectively resolved through drugs – but at HUGE cost.

Sleeping pills may have potential sedative and sleep-inducing effects, either as their main function or as a side effect, but none of them can stock the brain's energy reserve and induce a peaceful RESTORATIVE sleep like honey does.

The NHS spends an estimated £50 million every year on sleeping pills in an attempt to patch up what has become a very big problem. Considering that these synthetic drugs disrupt natural sleep patterns and invariably come with nasty side effects (which commonly include coordination problems, behavioural issues, confusion, headaches, dizziness, rashes) and the potential for addiction, modern medicine really isn't able to properly address the problem.

In October 2002, the English football team, who were due to play against Poland, were given caffeine pills before the game (a highly questionable strategy) to boost their energy levels. The game was postponed until the following day after a violent rain storm, and to counteract the stimulating effect of the caffeine, they were prescribed sleeping tablets. The result was disastrous. They performed woefully in a game that they were confident of winning (drawing one goal each) and were pilloried in the sporting press.

Although there is a certain questionable logic to giving caffeine tablets to perk up the sluggish players and then, when the match is postponed, suggesting sleeping tablets to wipe out the effect of the caffeine and help them sleep, the drug combination is, in fact, disastrous.

Both caffeine and sleeping pills block the smooth transportation of glucose into the muscles, and can result in slower reaction times, poor motor coordination and reduced running speeds. The players' blood would have been supercharged with energy, but not usable in the two organs where it was most required: the brain and muscle.

With such a double handicap inflicted on them by their advisors, the footballers can only be praised for playing out of their skins to secure a draw!

Chapter 3

HONEY – THE SWEET MIRACLE

Since the beginning of time, honey has been thought to have incredible healing, even mystical, properties and, although hardcore scientists have long been sceptical of its miraculous powers, in recent years serious scientific studies have started to uncover exciting confirmation of its goodness.

I am fascinated by honey and, after years of research, I am convinced this deliciously sweet superfood could hold the key to undoing some of the evil of the modern diet and lifestyles – it could even hold the key to long-term weight loss and good health.

Honey has always been one of mankind's most highly regarded foods. Until relatively recent times, it was man's only source of sweetness apart from fruit. Honey was rare and difficult – even dangerous – to get hold of.

In Spain, there are cave paintings of honey that date back 8,000 years and records show that the ancient Egyptians were avid honey eaters, as were the Greeks and Romans.

Honey has long been revered as more than just a source of food in a whole host of ancient religious writings. In fact, all of the great religions of the world seem to feature honey in their sacred texts.

In Hindu writings, honey features as one of the Five Elixirs of Immortality. When Buddha retired to the wilderness, a monkey brought him honey to eat. Likewise in Christianity, the New Testament describes John the Baptist as surviving in the wilderness on a diet of honey and locusts. The Jewish religious tradition regards honey as a symbol of the New Year and describes the Promised Land as 'flowing with milk and honey'. The Islamic religion has been especially interested in honey and its benefits. It is mentioned in the Qur'an:

'And thy Lord taught the bee to build its cells in hills, on trees and in (men's) habitations . . . there issues from within their bodies a drink of varying colours, wherein is healing for mankind. Verily in this is a Sign for those who give thought.' (Qur'an 16:68-9)

In addition, the Prophet referred at length to honey and bees in writings: It is reported by Al-Bukhari that a man came to the Prophet because his brother had a stomach disorder. The Prophet said, 'Let him drink honey.' The man returned a second time, complaining that no improvement happened in his brother's case, and again the Prophet responded, 'Let him drink honey.' The man returned again and said, 'I have done that, but to no avail.' Thereupon the Prophet responded, 'Allah has said the truth, but your brother's stomach has told a lie. Let him drink honey.' He drank it and was cured. (Al-Bukhari)

HONEY AND EXERCISE

For me, my intense interest in honey first began when I was working with my son, an exercise specialist, on a scientific project to try to find the best food and drink to maximize performance in high-level athletes.

I discovered research that indicates that the liver plays a crucial role in our ability to keep exercising for long periods of time – and found that honey has a very close and beneficial relationship with the liver.

After a meal, the food you eat is usually converted into glucose in the blood and sent off around the body. Some goes to the muscles to be held in glycogen stores there (ready to be called upon to fuel the muscle action when you are exercising) and some goes to the liver, where it is stored in special glycogen pockets.

The liver's glycogen stores seem to exist as a kind of 'grab-and-go' fuel supply for the brain, which it can plunder either during the night when we go for many hours without eating or during exercise, as blood glucose levels run low.

However, as muscle glycogen levels are run down (by exercise) the body 'borrows' from the brain's liver glycogen reserves.

Exercise specialists over the years have typically put all their refuelling focus on the glycogen stores in our muscles and I was hard pushed to spot any mention of the role of liver glycogen. In fact, as I researched further, I was amazed at how few experts seemed to understand that exercise will often deplete these liver reserves and so leave the brain with worryingly low supplies.

This is NOT a good idea! The brain is utterly dependent on the liver glycogen and simply cannot function effectively if it is worrying about its fuel supply. If your brain isn't working properly, you won't be going anywhere, let alone fast.

If your brain gets really hungry, as Paula Radcliffe most probably found during the 2004 Athens Olympics, it instigates collapse, and there's nothing you can do about it.

It occurred to me that many athletes and their coaches were just not aware of how critically important it is to ensure the liver's glycogen reserves are well stocked during and after exercise.

I can understand how it could have slipped their attention. Tests show that if you take blood from a collapsed athlete, their blood sugar levels will usually register as normal. This may seem counterintuitive, but it shows that the glycogen stores have been keeping their blood glucose levels topped up right to the point of collapse.

But if an athlete pushes themselves to the absolute limit, it means their exertions will have seriously plundered those glycogen reserves and left worryingly little for the brain. As the conductor of the body's orchestra, the brain has no option but to switch everything off and instigate collapse – it is the only way to stop the muscles sucking glucose out of the blood, and keep a little glucose left in the blood for itself.

With those crucial liver reserves in mind, we set out to test different types of food and drink that could swiftly and effectively replenish the liver's glycogen reserves.

Our tests with fructose-based drinks found that fruit sugar was better at restocking the liver during and after exercise than ordinary table sugar. We tried a sports drink made from honey powder and were astounded by its success. It seems there is something in honey that directs the sugars straight to the liver, and keeps the brain's fuel supply brilliantly topped up. This is not the case for sugar-based drinks.

We found honey (diluted in water) to be the perfect food for athletes competing in arduous triathlons and ironman events.

If you eat or drink honey before exercising, it swiftly restocks the glycogen stores without causing a blood sugar spike. This gives the body a steady supply of fuel and stops the brain worrying, which reduces fatigue and allows athletes to work harder and for longer periods of time.

Many athletes around the world now use honey (drinking honey in water either just before or during exercise) to boost their performance. In fact, Serbian tennis star Novak Djokovic admits in his autobiography that he enjoys 2 tablespoons of honey with his breakfast every morning before embarking on his arduous daily training regime.

But, sadly, the message hasn't filtered through to everyone. In 2002, the England football team were knocked out of the World Cup in Japan and Korea when their manager Sven-Göran Eriksson ordered the team chef to put Jaffa Cakes on the menu to fuel the players at half-time.

Although the high calorie content might have given the players an energy boost, their brains would have been relying on the liver's energy reserves to keep things ticking over mentally. A tough first half of play will have depleted those liver glycogen reserves, so by half-time it's very likely their brains were beginning to get a bit hungry.

Their hungry brains would have been forced to activate a stress response, releasing the hormone cortisol in an effort to get more fuel for the brain. But cortisol has many side effects, and one of them is that it slows the transfer of glucose into contracting muscles (so it can hang on to the glucose for itself!). This meant that although those half-time Jaffa Cakes would have sent blood sugar levels soaring, the glucose wouldn't have got to the players' muscles in anything like the speed or quantity needed, and wouldn't have restocked the liver's glycogen stores.

So by allowing his players to get brain hungry (or by failing to understand the importance of restocking their fuel reserves properly at half-time), Eriksson inadvertently slowed their reaction times – not a wise fuelling strategy in such an important competition.

Honey (dissolved in water and taken as a drink) would have given a far, far more effective half-time energy boost. It would have immediately targeted the players' livers, replenished their glycogen stores and ensured they were fit and alert and ready for the second half.

Very interestingly, we also found that if the athletes took honey at night, they slept better and their tired muscles appeared to recover more effectively.

We know that proper sleep requires sufficient fuel for the brain to keep ticking over effectively throughout the night. So, having watched the improved repair and recovery process that athletes enjoyed after a honey-fuelled sleep, I went on to investigate whether honey might be useful for ordinary night-time recovery in non-athletes, too.

My research has shown that 1 to 2 tablespoons of honey taken just before bed has exactly the same beneficial effect on non-athletes. It replenishes glycogen stores in the liver, which may be depleted after an early evening meal, and means the brain does not go hungry during the night and is perfectly comfortable choreographing the important process of repair and recovery, unfettered by stress or concerns about fuel supply.

THE AMAZING HONEY BEE

A foraging honey bee weighing less than half a gram may fly at 10 miles per hour for up to 10 miles. That's equivalent to a 12 stone (75kg) human travelling 1.5 million miles at 1.5 million miles per hour.

When worker bees set off on a mission to forage for nectar, they first load up with honey from the honeycombs in the hive as the fuel for their long flight. Their tiny bodies process the glucose from this honey and fuel their contracting muscles at a speed that is almost beyond scientific understanding.

HOW HONEY IS DIFFERENT FROM SUGAR

There is still quite a lot of misunderstanding about the differences between honey and sugar. Many people – even dietary experts – put the two in the same category. But honey is very different. It may be rich in sugars and would therefore be expected to function in a similar way to sugar, but the fascinating thing is, it doesn't.

Honey is created from sweet plant nectar, which bees ingest and then regurgitate several times. Bees act as a kind of natural processing plant for the honey. This regurgitation process is crucial, because after several regurgitations the honey becomes partially digested, and the action of the enzymes in the bee's digestive tract during this process performs a kind of metabolic miracle that explains how honey behaves completely differently from sugar.

When we eat something sweet – like a doughnut or a bar of chocolate – blood glucose levels will rise dramatically and swiftly. Some of this glucose will be directed to muscles and other organs, and a small quantity will go to the liver's glycogen stores. But insulin levels will rise dramatically as our body tries to deal with this sugary onslaught, and, as a direct consequence, much of the glucose will be carted off out of the way to be stored as fat around the body.

But drink a cup of tea sweetened with honey, or drizzle honey on yoghurt, and the sugars behave in a completely different way. In fact, tests show a spoonful of honey appears to *lower* blood sugar levels rather than raise them as sugar would (see box).

If you switch from sugar to honey in your diet, you will be better able to keep your insulin levels stable, and this is great news for your body and brain because, as I have mentioned earlier, insulin is the 'bad boy' hormone that causes weight gain, premature ageing, heart disease and dementia.

WHY HONEY DOESN'T RAISE BLOOD SUGAR LEVELS

When we eat honey, the sugar molecules are absorbed into our bloodstream, and they travel first to the liver. Here the fructose particles are extracted, converted to glucose, and tucked away into the liver's glycogen stores. The fructose also activates mechanisms that draw extra glucose into the liver, too. This means that the liver's glycogen stores get packed really tightly – much more effectively than they would when we eat ordinary sugars, and this makes it a more stable store of glycogen than one created from sugar alone.

Because the sugars are taken out of the blood and so swiftly stored in the liver, the body doesn't get the chance to register a blood sugar spike, and doesn't have to instruct the release of such quantities of insulin.

Furthermore, if your muscles run out of fuel and start trying to plunder the liver's glycogen reserves, honey seems to be able to hang on to that glycogen and hold it back for the brain's use only. The fructose in honey appears to exert some kind of control over the enzyme that would normally trigger the release of glucose from the liver's glycogen stores on demand.

This amazing process ONLY works when the fructose comes from honey. It certainly doesn't work if you eat high fructose corn syrup (the modern fructose derivative found in thousands of modern processed foods) or other refined sugars.

HONEY CURES CRAVINGS

After a meal, it is very important that any glucose in your food be sent to the liver to be stored in the glycogen reserves, so that it is available as a fuel supply for the brain between meals and during the night.

But if you've eaten a high-sugar meal (with NO honey), the huge surge of glucose will increase the amount of sugar in your blood and could cause the iPump to short-circuit, slowing the uptake of glucose by the brain and triggering the stress response, which puts the body into emergency mode.

If you had sweetened your meal with honey, things might have been very different. Honey's sugars would be directed straight to replenish the liver's glycogen reserves, there would be no blood sugar rush, and the iPump would continue operating just as it should.

Honey also appears to protect the liver against harmful toxins and has some kind of role to play in protecting it from what scientists call 'oxidative damage'. This is all part of daily wear and tear for the liver cells, as they bear the brunt of the corrosive effects of sugars and oxygen.

The beneficial role honey takes in protecting the liver like this has been shown to help keep blood glucose levels throughout the body steady. This increases the chance that the iPump will continue to function normally (or start to function normally if it has been tripped by a sugar onslaught), meaning the brain WON'T get hungry and won't need to send out furious appetite signals (in the form of those impossible-to-resist cravings).

In the 1960s, a Mexican researcher, Mauricio Russek, suggested that the liver could have some kind of role to play in appetite control, but his work was ignored and forgotten. However, I think

Russek could have been way ahead of his time. His studies were able to show that the liver contains special receptors that are extremely sensitive to glucose. He also showed that when the liver's glycogen stores are replenished, our appetite tends to be reduced.

This backs up the Honey Diet philosophy that hunger is actually driven by the brain seeking new sources of energy (and not by a grumbling stomach looking for more food).

Recent work by Jean-Marc Lavoie in Montreal shows that the liver releases a signal to warn the brain if its glycogen stores are running low, so causing the brain to trigger the stress response and stimulate appetite. This confirms that Russek was on the right track.

If the liver is always well stocked, the brain can relax and reduce the stress reaction (so no more cravings).

Hunger and stress cause confusion and use up vital brain energy supplies, but if you sweeten your food with honey you should find that during the day you feel sharper and more mentally focussed. At night, you'll sleep better, and you'll wake up in the morning feeling rested because your body and brain have been doing all the recovery and repair they should, unhindered by pesky stress hormones swimming around.

If you respond to a massive chocolate craving by eating chocolate (as your body demands) you will only overload the body with glucose, suppress the iPump and reactivate the stress and appetite response further.

But if you respond to a craving by eating honey, the honey sugars will be stored and, because the glucose is not swimming around in the blood, you reduce both your glucose and insulin load, keep your iPump happy, the brain happy and so reduce any impulse to eat.

Honey immediately silences cravings.

CASE STUDY

Karen, 42, a shop assistant from Macclesfield, lost half a stone (3kg) in 5 weeks on the Honey Diet. She says:

'I've tried so many different diets, but this is the only one I can honestly say I've enjoyed. The honey drink before bed is just perfect for me. I find it somehow comforting – it's a real treat, and not the sort of thing I'd expect on a weight-loss diet. I'm absolutely convinced the honey drink allows me to sleep more soundly, and I wake up determined to keep my sugar addiction under control for the rest of the day. I've noticed a real reduction in the cravings that used to drive me wild. If I do get a craving for something sweet, I know a cup of tea with a teaspoon of honey, or a pot of natural yoghurt with a bit of honey stirred in, will do the trick.'

HONEY AS EXERCISE FUEL

Honey is a high-octane fuel and perfect for fuelling both muscles and the brain during exercise – it restocks the liver, stops the brain worrying that its supplies might run out, and therefore allows the brain to release extra glucose into contracting muscles.

Here's how to use honey in sport:

1. Fifteen minutes before a 90-minute workout, take 2 tablespoons of honey dissolved in water
2. During the workout, take 6 to 8 tablespoons in 1 litre water (flavour it with a splash of natural fruit juice if you prefer)

3. After exercising, have a small snack (such as a mixed honey/grain bar) and then follow your Honey Diet regime

4. Your next meal should be high in protein, but have some extra carbohydrate to replenish any lost muscle glycogen

5. Always take honey before you go to bed to replenish your liver's glycogen reserves and ensure your muscles recover – and you burn the body fat you may have thought that you were burning during the workout

HONEY'S OTHER SECRET POWERS

Clearly the particular sugars in honey have a profound influence on the way in which we metabolize it, but there is much, much more to honey than merely its sugar content.

Honey is so intricate and complex in its construction that all attempts by scientists to mimic its qualities have so far failed. Dr Noori Al-Waili, a specialist in life support technologies in New York, has shown in studies that a solution containing the same ratio of sugars as honey cannot mimic the many metabolic benefits of honey in any way.

This is because every drop of honey is packed with up to two hundred beneficial bionutrients such as vitamins, minerals, amino acids, bioflavonoids (plant molecules that are anti-diabetic), disease-fighting antioxidants, organic acids, monosaccharides and oligosaccharides (sugars) and numerous enzymes.

Each of these two hundred special ingredients is there for a precise reason linked to a bee's survival, and they play a vital part and have a major influence on honey's health-giving properties.

A tablespoon of honey might contain a similar sugar profile

as a medium-sized apple or a portion of broccoli, but it is the additional nutrients that really set it apart.

The reason honey bees can process such colossal quantities of glucose, which should, in theory, shut down their delicate brains, is because of the many bioactive nutrients that protect the brain's function as they fly.

Although honey's unique ability to lower and stabilize blood glucose concentration is currently not fully understood, it is clear that ordinary refined carbohydrates and sugars contain none of these natural nutrients.

HONEY BEATS STRESS – THE HIDDEN DIVIDEND

One system that is never mentioned in scientific papers is honey's role in stress management. By ensuring a steady supply of energy to the brain, honey stops the brain triggering the stress reaction. This makes it a potent anti-stress food.

HONEY AND DIABETES

Any diabetic will tell you that sugar is the last thing they need in their diet, and honey is just as bad, but I think – certainly in the case of people with type 2 diabetes – they are wrong.

Studies show that honey improves the anti-diabetic action of diabetic medication and I am convinced that diabetics can safely use honey in place of any other sweetener in their diet.

Two well-known anti-diabetic medications used by people with type 2 diabetes are glibenclamide and metformin. A

Malaysian study in 2011 showed that when combined with either of these drugs, honey can improve glucose control (admittedly in rats) by as much as 30 per cent.

Honey has been shown to kill off the bacterium that causes gastric and duodenal ulcers and lesions (*Helicobacter pylori*), which means it could help reduce the risk of diabetes. The wrong bacteria in the gut can impair our ability to control the absorption of sugars (resulting in sudden spikes and surges). Honey seems to protect the gut lining, killing off the most damaging bacterium, too.

The clever thing is honey is great at improving the levels of friendly bacteria in the gut (such as bifido), and these bacteria are now known to have a positive influence in diabetes by improving glucose control and insulin function.

WARNING: If you have diabetes (either type 1 or type 2) talk to your GP or specialist before making any dietary changes.

HONEY AS A HANGOVER REMEDY

When we drink more than a few glasses of wine or have three or four pints on a night out, the alcohol will start to cause problems for our body and brain.

Alcohol suppresses the iPump in the same way that excess sugar does, by suppressing the enzyme that should be driving the pump. This, as we know, means that the glucose supply to the brain becomes compromised.

The reason why alcohol causes dehydration is because it acts as a diuretic (it causes water to be leached from the cells) but, additionally, if glucose cannot cross over into the brain neither can water, and glucose entry to the brain normally carries water with it by osmosis.

So when we drink excessively, our brain will become hungry AND dehydrated. It's a recipe for disaster!

If you've enjoyed a few drinks the previous night, you'll know the fuggy-headed, mini-hangover feeling the following morning. This happens because alcohol pushes your blood glucose levels down during the night as it depletes the liver and suppresses the iPump – a double whammy that leaves the brain short of energy. The hungry brain, forced to exist on insufficient fuel, gradually slows down (ever wondered why under the influence of alcohol we become stupid, uninhibited and unsteady on our feet?). If the stress release continues, the brain triggers the release of the hormone glucagon, which can make us feel nauseated and we may even vomit.

But while this is going on, the liver's glycogen reserves remain depleted, driving the stress hormones higher and higher and causing physiological and psychological havoc.

The brain will be totally focussed on one question: to save its life and get glucose into the liver and blood – it cannot concentrate on work or on intellectual matters. The glucose deprivation and dehydration in the brain go a long way to explain why we can behave so stupidly when we're drunk.

Such is the devastating impact on the brain that if we were to keep on drinking without restraint, we would eventually fall into a coma.

It is interesting to note that when paramedics attend a comatose drunk, they usually inject glucagon to trigger the release of any glucose that might be left in the liver as a swift way to get fuel to the poor brain. If this doesn't work, they set up a glucose drip to save the brain and therefore life.

Honey's action on the iPump and beneficial effect on the liver make it an excellent antidote to alcohol. It effectively protects the liver from alcohol-induced damage by recycling the alcohol detoxifying enzyme (alcohol dehydrogenase) and replenishing the liver's glycogen stores.

Honey naturally improves the action of the iPump and, in so doing, ensures a good reserve supply of energy for the brain after a big night out. Because it promotes the transfer of glucose into the brain, honey also improves water transport into the brain (water naturally accompanies the glucose), so reducing the dehydrating effects of alcohol consumption more effectively than drinking pints of water would.

Honey also suppresses the hormone glucagon, which would normally cause post-drinking nausea.

So taking honey before and after alcohol is a must. Take 1 tablespoon before you go out, 1 before bed, and 2 to 3 teaspoons first thing in the morning, either on wholemeal toast, in yoghurt or just neat, on a spoon.

CASE STUDY

Helen, 47, from Buckinghamshire.

'My favourite hangover remedy has always been a couple of painkillers, a Diet Coke and a packet of crisps, then lots of sweet foods all day to keep my energy levels up. But a friend recommended honey, so after a big wine-fuelled party recently, I switched my night-time hangover-preventing pint of water for a hot honey drink. In the morning I sipped a cup of hot water with honey when I woke up instead of my usual cup of tea. I have to admit I was pretty impressed with the impact. I quickly felt lucid and almost normal, mentally, and I was able to stick

to healthy eating for the rest of the day rather than being drawn to unhealthy stodge and puddings.'

MANUKA HONEY OR ANY HONEY?

Manuka honey, which comes from New Zealand, is made by bees taking nectar from the manuka (or tea) tree. It tends to be much darker in colour than other honeys, with a distinctive taste and – often – a high price tag.

The honey has an incredibly high concentration of a substance called methylglyoxal, which is believed to give Manuka honey potent antibacterial, antiviral and antifungal properties.

These qualities make Manuka honey potentially very interesting as an alternative treatment for a variety of ailments, and I am all in favour of continued research into its purported benefits. However, there is probably no need to pay Manuka honey prices to enjoy the health benefits of honey.

My advice is to buy honey from a local beekeeper if you can, but otherwise use a retailer you trust. It can be hard, honeycombed or runny, just as long as you are confident about its quality.

Some budget honeys can be adulterated (augmented with sugar syrup), so be wary of cheap brands and always buy the best you can afford.

WARNING – DON'T EAT TOO MUCH HONEY!

Such are the health benefits of honey it might be tempting to throw caution to the winds and eat or drink limitless quantities of the stuff. But this is not a great idea!

Start your day with 1 to 2 teaspoons of honey in hot water to prime your liver (getting the glycogen stores ready to take on board the contents of your breakfast), add honey to your yoghurts, drinks and fruits throughout the day, and end the day with a late-night honey drink.

But don't forget that honey is a source of calories (22 calories per teaspoon, 64 calories in a tablespoon), which can mount up if you go crazy for the stuff.

If you eat more honey than your liver's glycogen stores need (around 2 tablespoons at any one time), the rest will stay in circulation and will inevitably raise blood sugar levels and insulin levels. A real excess of honey could even be enough to trigger the iPump, which would go against everything you are hoping to achieve.

Honey should not be fed to infants below one year old, due to a small risk of botulism – their immune systems are not fully developed at that age, and the spores can find their way into some foods, of which honey is one.

Chapter 4

HOW THE HONEY DIET WORKS

It is quite clear that the food we eat has a huge impact on our health and most of us have slipped into bad eating habits that are making us ill.

I am convinced that to get the body into a state of balance where it functions exactly as it should – without gaining weight or accelerating ageing or disease – we need to feed our body and brain a simple, basic, healthy diet.

If your body is getting the nutrients it needs, without having to somehow deal with the never-ending barrage of sugar, refined carbohydrates and junk food, it will have a much better chance of functioning as it is supposed to.

The benefits of the Honey Diet are so far-reaching, and so incredible, they should be available to everyone, regardless of whether or not you want to lose weight. So, with this in mind, I have divided the diet into two phases: phase 1 and phase 2.

Phase 1 of the Honey Diet offers a quick, simple and healthy dietary regime suitable for everyone. It's a great honey-based starting point and a safe plan if you just want to make the most of all the health-giving properties of honey.

The best way to eat in phase 1 is quite simply to choose simple, fresh foods and cut out junk. If you banish sugar, use honey as your only sweetener and commit to a regular dose of honey before bed each night, you will be giving your body the best possible chance of beating disease, staying youthful and losing weight.

For many people, these simple dietary changes will be enough to improve health forever. You will be ensuring your delicate brain cells get exactly the right mix of high-octane fuel throughout the day and, crucially, throughout the night, so all the repair and recovery happens exactly as it should. You'll notice your concentration improves, your memory and your ability to focus. You will be reducing your risk of dementia and Alzheimer's. Your happy brain will have no need to send out the stress signals that, over time, wreak havoc on every single cell in your body. So you will suffer fewer colds and infections, and enjoy a dramatically reduced risk of serious illnesses – even heart disease. You will be sleeping better and, if you are carrying a few extra pounds, you should find your waist slims down as your body begins to burn fat efficiently while you sleep at night.

The basic rules to follow are outlined in phase 1 of the Honey Diet below. The measures are simple and delicious and you should find it easy to adapt the way you eat. And the results will be so swift and so dramatic that you'll make sure there is always honey in the kitchen cupboard. You won't ever want to go back to your old ways of eating again.

However, if you have more than a stone of weight to lose, and slenderness is your ultimate goal, move on to phase 2 of the diet as soon as you have grasped the principles of phase 1. Phase 2 incorporates additional dietary changes – such as switching to wholemeal carbohydrates and getting into the habit of one no-carb day each week, which will further harness the power of honey to ensure that excess pounds swiftly and effort-lessly fall away.

If you have tried diets in the past and have either struggled to stick with them or found you lost weight but then regained it, I can reassure you that the Honey Diet is very different.

This plan works in harmony with your body, completely changing the chemical cascade that causes cravings and drives every sweet indulgence straight to your fat stores. So from the minute you commit to the Honey Diet, you will regain control over what and when you eat and you will burn fat like never before.

If you follow the rules of phase 2 and your body is working as it really should, you can expect to lose 3lb a week and as much as a stone in a month. But you won't go hungry, or have to fork out on expensive diet foods. You can enjoy proper deli-cious family meals, snacks and treats – including puddings, bread, muffins, even biscuits.

The Honey Diet is so easy and so delicious that it will become a way of eating for life. You will not only get slim and stay slim forever, but you will be healthier than you have ever been before.

FOLLOW THE HONEY DIET AND YOUR BODY CAN EXPECT THESE CHANGES

1. No more surges and spikes in blood sugar mean your body won't have to pump out huge quantities of insulin in its attempts to deal with the sugar overload – so less sugar in your diet is turned to BODY FAT
2. Your iPump won't be tripped by dietary sugar surges and will function as it should, ensuring a steady fuel supply to the brain

3. With a secure fuel supply, your brain cells won't get hungry, so won't pump out appetite-stimulating stress hormones, which would drive you to eat high-sugar foods. This means NO MORE CRAVINGS

4. Without those hungry-brain stress hormones, your body's daily stress load (and the damage it causes) will be dramatically reduced.

5. With your iPump working well, there's no hungry-brain stress hormones to keep you awake so you will SLEEP WELL

6. Because you are sleeping well, there will be nothing to stop your body going into repair and recovery mode at night – the process that BURNS FAT as you sleep

THE HONEY DIET – PHASE I

RULE NUMBER I: SWITCH SUGAR FOR HONEY

The first, and most important, step you can take towards great health is to cut all sugar and artificial sweeteners out of your life. There is absolutely no doubt in my mind that sugar is a great big modern evil that wreaks havoc on our bodies and our brain.

It's not just a question of sprinkling a little less sugar into your coffee or tea or switching to water when you're thirsty instead of a full-sugar or no-sugar fizzy drink. If you want to get the full health and weight-loss benefits from the Honey Diet, you really should be watching out for the stealth sugar that manufacturers add to virtually EVERYTHING you eat.

In the UK we swallow a worrying 46 teaspoons of sugar a day – much of that without even realizing. Partly because it makes cheap food and low-fat food taste so much better, so boosting consumption and therefore sales, sugar is added to a hideously long list of foods – both sweet and savoury.

The worst offenders are processed food, particularly ready meals and cereals. A bowl of Coco Pops, for instance, can contain nearly 7 teaspoons of sugar; a muffin with your morning coffee will add another 6 teaspoons; you might find 5 teaspoons in your pizza; 9 in a fizzy drink and as much as 9 in a ready meal such as sweet-and-sour chicken.

Most of the sugar we eat is rushed out of our blood and converted as quickly as possible into body fat (it's the best way the body knows of saving the energy in case we need it in the future). Fat in the diet is always blamed for our podgy thighs, bingo wings or bulging waistlines, but every 1g of sugar we eat becomes 2g of fat. So every spoonful of sugar you say no to means a potential 10g of fat you won't be adding to your waistline!

If you eat real food, simple food, and banish the white stuff from your life, you will be taking the best possible step for your future health.

Cutting out sugar is a very big step to take, and one that you might need to ease into gradually. But over time, your taste buds will change and you won't miss it.

The big bonus of the Honey Diet is that you don't have to deny yourself sweetness completely. You can quite simply replace all the sugar in your diet with honey. This is the key to cutting out cravings. Once you make the switch from sugar to honey, you should be free of the tyranny of the 'munchies' or late-night urges for chocolate.

Although many nutritionists might tell you honey is no better than sugar, the science proves otherwise. Our bodies metabolize honey in a completely different way to sugar, and the hundreds of micronutrients in every teaspoon of honey, although micro-scopic, dramatically change the way the substance reacts in our digestive system.

So go ahead and use honey in tea or coffee, in cakes and biscuits (see the recipes in chapter 6), on cereal, in cooking . . . its uses are endless, and you can be quietly confident that not only are you getting a little sweetness in your life, but you are likely to be doing yourself a lot of good at the same time.

RULE NUMBER 2: HAVE A HONEY DRINK EVERY NIGHT BEFORE BED

Every night, about 30 minutes before you go to bed, dissolve 1 to 2 tablespoons (around 50g) of honey in a cup of boiling water and sip this as your bedtime drink.

My research has shown that this is exactly the right amount of honey to perfectly stock up the glycogen reserves in the liver, which ensures your brain has enough fuel to last the night. This means your brain will not need to pump out damaging stress hormones in its quest for fuel, and the repair and recovery process that should be going on at night (which burns lots of lovely body fat as it does so) can continue unimpaired.

If your iPump has been tripped by too much sugar and refined carbohydrates during the day, just 50g of honey before bed is enough to un-trip that switch and set you on the right path for a really great night's fat-burning sleep.

RULE NUMBER 3: NO MORE JUNK FOOD

Cut all processed food out of your diet.

This means you need to take a seriously long look at any food you eat that comes in a packet or from a takeaway.

Honey can do a lot of the good work in your body, but make life a bit easier for yourself by avoiding the empty calories, and potential damage, that artificial and processed foods provide, and commit to feeding your body the highest-octane fuel you can.

If you are going to take the Honey Diet seriously, you'll have to avoid crisps, fizzy drinks (even diet drinks), sweets/chocolate, fried foods, processed foods (anything in a packet), takeaways, cakes and pastries. I'm not saying this is going to be easy at first, but the health benefits are enormous.

If you need a snack, have a small handful of nuts. If you need something sweet, spread honey on toast or a cracker or add a teaspoon to a small tub of natural yoghurt.

Once the Honey Diet rules become second nature and you start to notice the dramatic improvements in your mental and physical health, you will find it impossible to comprehend how you were once able to eat so much pappy, artificial food pumped with chemicals. From now on, the odd slip won't do you too much harm, but it makes sense to avoid rubbish food if you can and to give your body – and brain – the best possible chance of working at their best.

RULE NUMBER 4: ENJOY A GOOD BREAKFAST

These days, the typical British breakfast has become a cup of tea or coffee with a muffin on the run or a bowl of sweetened cereal – which couldn't be more unhealthy!

The caffeine hit from an early morning cuppa only gets your stress hormones fired up, while the rush of unrefined sugar from a bowl of cereal or a muffin will start your day with a massive sugar rush, which forces the body to pump out insulin. This means each day begins in fat-storing mode and you set yourself up for an inevitable sugar crash and impossible-to-resist sugar cravings around mid-morning.

Skipping breakfast is even worse – it is a known route to weight gain.

If you are one of the many people who just can't stomach the idea of breakfast in the morning, it could be a sign that your brain got hungry in the night. Your hungry brain may have been pumping out certain stress hormones, which trigger feelings of nausea (it is the hormone that triggers morning sickness in pregnant women).

However, if you do force yourself to eat a piece of toast, you will normally find you feel better because the food replenishes the liver's glycogen stores and stabilizes blood sugar levels, so you stop releasing the nauseating hormones and start to feel more normal. Toast with honey would be even better!

On the Honey Diet, we recommend starting the day with a teaspoon or two of honey dissolved in hot water. This small spike of glucose will prime your liver's glycogen stores ready for breakfast. Then your ideal Honey Diet breakfast would combine protein (eggs, bacon, yoghurt, cheese, ham) with some wholemeal carbohydrates – and honey (see chapter 6 for some breakfast ideas).

RULE NUMBER 5: ENJOY UNLIMITED SALAD AND VEGETABLES

Don't hold back on the number and variety of vegetables and salads in your diet. Vegetables are high in fibre as well as vitamins, so aim for six to nine portions a day if you can. You owe it to your body and your health.

Most salad and vegetables contain 'phyto' (or plant) nutrients, which are now known to be essential for good health – physical and mental. For instance, lycopene (found in tomatoes, melons, red peppers, red onions and radicchio) has been shown to protect against cancer, particularly prostate cancer. Garlic and leeks contain a compound called allicin, which promotes heart health, and salicylates, which have strong anti-inflammatory and anti-oxidative properties (which is good because inflammation is at the root of most degenerative diseases, including brain diseases such as Alzheimer's).

Fresh food is higher in nutrients, so aim for seasonal and locally grown or even frozen – food that is picked and immediately frozen is sometimes better than something that has been languishing on a supermarket shelf for weeks.

RULE NUMBER 6: FULL-FAT DAIRY PRODUCTS ARE OK

There is a massive craze for reduced-fat, even 0% fat, dairy products, but I think that's a false saving. Stripping the fat out of dairy products invariably means adding in gelling agents, bulking agents, sweeteners or sugars to make the resulting concoction palatable.

Studies have shown that full-fat yoghurt is far more satisfying than reduced-fat (it keeps you feeling fuller for longer) and the best product you could choose is natural bio-yoghurt – delicious with a little added honey.

Dairy products are a really important source of calcium, plus they can aid weight loss (even full-fat dairy products can). Milk protein seems to be particularly filling and there's evidence that the calcium in dairy foods acts almost like a detergent, grabbing fat before it can be absorbed. It's only a small effect, but it probably amounts to around 45 calories a day that you don't have to lose elsewhere in your diet. On top of that, dairy is a rich source of calcium, which may benefit blood pressure and is vital for bone health.

But don't go crazy. If you overdo the full-fat dairy products, the calories will start to add up. Many people actually prefer the taste of semi-skimmed to full-fat milk, but stop wasting your money on sickly sweet, pappy diet yoghurts and introduce yourself to the glorious rich, creamy taste of proper natural live yoghurt – in moderation!

This means no more than one small pot of yoghurt or cottage cheese, one matchbox-size piece of cheese (buy mature cheese, which packs more flavour for fewer calories) and up to 500ml milk per day.

RULE NUMBER 7: DRINK LOTS OF WATER

Your body needs water to function properly, but most of us don't drink enough. Instead of fruit juice, fizzy drinks (sugar-packed or 'diet'), drink more water. Aim for eight large glasses a day.

On the Honey Diet, coffee and tea are allowed, but try not to drink more than six cups a day and, ideally, not before breakfast (no sugar – add honey if desired).

THE HONEY DIET – PHASE 2

For some people, phase 1 of the Honey Diet will be extremely easy – more of a reminder about healthy eating habits than a dramatic dietary change. But others may take longer to adapt. If your diet has become reliant on high-sugar convenience foods, you may find it takes a few weeks before you feel able to drop sugar and abandon junk food forever.

Because of the way the Honey Diet deals with cravings, you should find that even on phase 1 your eating patterns are much easier to control, and because the diet accelerates fat burning at night, you will start slimming down and losing any excess pounds immediately.

However, any serious weight-loss regime requires more stringent measures and phase 2 of the diet is carefully calculated to maximize weight loss while harnessing all the health benefits of honey.

You may choose to spend a few days, or even weeks, on phase 1 of the diet to get used to life without sugar or junk food before you move on to the weight-loss section of the diet. However, if you are keen to get cracking, there is nothing stopping you from throwing yourself right in straight away. Simply combine the measures in phase 1 and phase 2, and get started right now.

Continue following the rules from phase 1:

RULE NUMBER 1: SWITCH SUGAR FOR HONEY

RULE NUMBER 2: HAVE A HONEY DRINK EVERY NIGHT BEFORE BED

RULE NUMBER 3: NO MORE JUNK FOOD

RULE NUMBER 4: ENJOY A GOOD BREAKFAST

RULE NUMBER 5: ENJOY UNLIMITED SALAD AND VEGETABLES

RULE NUMBER 6: FULL-FAT DAIRY PRODUCTS ARE OK

RULE NUMBER 7: DRINK LOTS OF WATER

and combine with the new rules for phase 2:

RULE NUMBER 8: ONE NO-CARB DAY EACH WEEK

There have been lots of exciting studies in recent years about the benefits – in terms of health AND weight loss – of intermittent dieting, and I am convinced that giving your body a break from carbohydrates one day a week will reap dividends on both counts.

If you spend just one day steering clear of ALL forms of bread, pasta, flour (cakes, biscuits etc), potatoes, rice and cereal, you will reduce your insulin levels dramatically.

Most of us have far too much insulin washing around in our bodies, and if you're overweight, there's a strong chance you have a condition called insulin resistance. This means your cells are so tired of the insulin onslaught they no longer react or respond to insulin as they should. Your body has no option but to pump out yet more insulin in its attempt to get a response. Insulin resistance means your body could be trying to cope with vast quantities of the hormone. Numerous studies are now pointing at insulin as the possible 'bad guy' behind not only diabetes, but also heart disease and many cancers.

Cutting out carbohydrates just one day each week should be enough to reset your iPump if it has become accustomed to being suppressed, and should set you up with lower insulin levels for the rest of the week – as long as you stick to the other Honey Diet rules and keep away from sugar as much as you possibly can.

A no-carb day can take a little getting used to, but make it a habit on a certain day of the week and stick to it. You shouldn't feel hungry if you eat plenty of protein (lean meat, fish, dairy products such as yoghurt and cottage cheese, or vegetarian protein substitutes such as tofu or Quorn) and enjoy salads and plenty (unlimited) low-carbohydrate vegetables (that's everything apart from bulky vegetables like carrots, swede, parsnips and potatoes, plus peas and sweet corn).

This simple rule probably works best if you make your no-carb day the same day each week – say Monday. Kick off each week with a clean slate and you are more likely to stick to a healthy diet for the rest of the week, and keep your iPump functioning optimally.

RULE NUMBER 9: SWITCH TO BROWN CARBOHYDRATES (AND NOT TOO MANY)

We have all become accustomed to white refined flour, white pasta and white rice, and all junk and processed food is usually highly refined. It is cheaper, easier to manufacture and has a longer shelf life – it's no wonder the big food manufacturers are so keen for you to eat the stuff.

But white flour contains very few nutrients and is swiftly absorbed by the body, causing blood sugar spikes (and a rush of insulin). Wholemeal bread, pasta and brown rice are full of fibre, which means not only are they good for your digestion, but they take longer for your body to process, which means you'll feel fuller for longer. A bowl of white pasta is converted instantly into a bowl of white sugar inside you. Wholemeal pasta is completely different. You are less likely to get blood sugar surges and your insulin levels are more likely to remain stable.

If your iPump is suppressed, and your body is pumping out appetite hormones, you'll find it much more difficult to overeat if you've only got wholemeal carbohydrates in the kitchen.

There are additional health benefits to be had, too. Wholemeal carbs are rich in essential nutrients, they will help you feel full and they are an essential part of a good, healthy, balanced diet. They are also high in insoluble fibre, which prevents constipation and bowel problems, and have a higher nutritional content than white grains because they retain the outer layers of the grain where most of the nutrients are found. Fibre also keeps you feeling full for longer, reducing the desire for sugary foods.

Along with a rising number of health experts, I don't agree with the distribution of foods on the Government's 'eatwell' plate. The official dietary recommendations issued by the Government Food Standards Agency are that one third of all your meals should be made up of starchy foods. In my opinion, that's far too much. If you want to balance your insulin levels (and, let's be frank, that's got to be a big dietary health concern), you need to cut that back and make wholegrain carbohydrates take up less than a quarter of your plate at any meal.

Protein and vegetables should become the new-found heroes on your plate.

On phase 2 of the diet, try to stick to no more than two slices of wholemeal bread a day and no more than five to six oatcakes, rice cakes or Ryvita a day. So if you have toast for breakfast, try to think about something like soup or a big salad, rather than a sandwich, for lunch.

When you put carbohydrates like pasta or rice on your plate, serve yourself a fist-sized portion – no larger. A plate piled high with steaming pasta or rice will not help you lose weight. You can fill up more healthily instead by switching bread, potatoes or rice for a portion of starchy vegetables like sweet potato (no more than one a day), butternut squash, parsnips and carrots, plus beans (aduki, cannellini, kidney etc) or lentils. Try using beans (cannellini beans, butter beans, kidney beans) to bulk out a meal instead of potatoes or bread and, as frequently as possible, as a healthier source of protein in place of meat or eggs. Split peas, broad beans, chickpeas and lentils are rich in soluble fibre, proteins, minerals and vitamins. As a health bonus, soluble fibre binds with bile salts from the liver, preventing cholesterol being absorbed and so reducing risks for heart disease, stroke and obesity. They are more nutrient-packed and the extra fibre means your body takes longer to metabolize them and your blood sugar levels remain more stable.

Cutting down on carbohydrates on 6 days a week shouldn't leave you feeling hungry as long as you are getting enough protein into every meal. It's just a question of changing the emphasis from 'carbs with everything' to 'carbs on the side', and this may take a little time to get used to.

It may sound tough, but it is a really good idea, if you are serious about losing weight, to ban potatoes completely – in all forms from crisps to chips, to mash to baked. Potatoes burn so quickly in the body's furnace and are notorious for sending insulin levels shooting. It's easy to substitute other root vegetables instead and serve roasted root vegetables with a meal or mashed butternut squash, sweet potatoes, celeriac or swede. They provide filling bulk, plus nutrients, that potatoes simply can't offer.

Psychologists have found that sticking to diet rules is easier if you can apply one simple blanket ruling. Try 'no potatoes, at all, ever'. It is an easier rule to stick to than a more nebulous ruling such as 'no chips, crisps or roast potatoes and only mashed or boiled in moderation'.

RULE NUMBER 10: INCLUDE PROTEIN IN EVERY MEAL OR SNACK

Ensuring you have at least SOME protein in every meal will keep you feeling fuller for longer and prevent dangerous blood sugar spikes, which further protects you from cravings. Protein tends to be filling (research shows our body will keep telling us we are hungry until we've eaten enough protein) and helps maintain muscle strength.

If you are hoping to lose weight, it's a good idea to opt for lean protein wherever possible to keep calorie intake down. So opt for chicken (no skin), pork (fat trimmed), beef (as steak or 5% fat mince), eggs, lamb (trim and slow cook to allow excess fat to drain), but also don't forget excellent vegetable sources of protein like hummus, peanut butter and the huge assortment of lentils, beans and pulses.

Fish is an important addition to phase 2 of the Honey Diet. It is recommended in phase 1, but compulsory in phase 2 of a healthy Honey Diet. Aim to eat as many as four portions of fish a week, of which two portions are oily fish such as sardines, salmon, tuna and anchovies, which are rich in health-giving omega-3 fatty acids. These help to reduce dangerous blood fats (triglycerides), which are a major factor in heart disease, and also appear to protect against heart attack by reducing blood pressure and helping to prevent blood platelets from clotting. Fatty acids have an anti-inflammatory effect, protecting not only against cancer but inflammatory conditions such as rheumatoid arthritis.

All fish is considered a good low-fat source of protein (as long as it's not deep-fried in batter or drowned in a creamy sauce). Fresh fish is best, and the fresher the better as the omega-3 diminishes with age (and if fish isn't efficiently frozen). But if you can't get fresh, canned salmon, mackerel, pilchards and sardines all contain equivalent omega-3s.

Unfortunately, tuna loses much of its omega-3 benefit when canned (because the heating process removes much of the fat). Smoked fish loses none of its fatty acids, but watch out for the high salt content, particularly in kippers – stick to one portion per week.

For breakfast, protein can take the form of eggs, bacon, peanut butter and yoghurt. For lunch, add tuna, eggs, ham or pulses to a salad. And for dinner, try to include a protein portion roughly the size of the palm of your hand.

RULE NUMBER 11: NO MORE THAN TWO PIECES OF FRUIT (NOT JUICE) PER DAY

Fruit is packed with antioxidants, but it can also be high in sugars, so you might struggle to lose weight if you eat more than two servings per day (one serving is an apple, banana or orange or a small bowl of berries). When choosing fruit, try to favour low-carbohydrate fruit like berries or rhubarb, certainly on your no-carb day. These are relatively high in fibre and nutrients in relation to sugars, so they are less likely to cause a blood sugar spike.

Fruit is always better eaten than drunk as juice or mashed into a smoothie. The problem with fruit juice is the way it delivers a rush of fruit sugar straight into your bloodstream, triggering a surge in unhealthy insulin and maximizing the probability that the sugar will be stored somewhere on your hips or waist as fat. When we eat an orange or an apple, the fibre it contains forms a protective layer that acts as a barrier to the intestine. This slows the absorption of sugar, so the liver has a chance to catch up. For instance, 500ml of fresh orange juice contains 51g of sugar – the same as thirteen McVitie's Hobnob biscuits, while 250ml of grape juice has as much sugar as four glazed doughnuts. Try carrot or vegetable juice instead.

Chapter 5

MAKING THE HONEY DIET
WORK FOR YOU

The Honey Diet is refreshingly simple. It is about good, healthy eating, with honey at its heart. I firmly believe everyone, whatever their age and state of health, will benefit from taking on board the Honey Diet principles.

It is so wonderfully straightforward. You don't have to go on a drastic calorie-counted diet. No need to rush out and buy cupboards full of expensive diet products – the only investment you'll need to make is to buy a large jar of honey. And, unlike so many draconian diet plans, you won't have to subject yourself to a routine of gritty brown foods with no taste and no sweetness in your life.

If you have embarked on phase 1 of the Honey Diet (as outlined in chapter 4), you will be enjoying the full range of health benefits and can bask in the knowledge that your body is now efficiently burning fat at night. Phase 1 should be enough to kick-start your iPump if it hasn't been working properly, reduce the levels of destructive stress hormones swimming around your body and ensure you sleep soundly at night. And, as I explained in previous pages, a good night's sleep means you should be burning fat while you are lying there doing absolutely nothing!

Phase 2 will require a little more commitment, but you will see your reward on the scales as soon as the end of the first week. By cutting back on carbohydrates, switching from all-white to wholemeal, and getting into the habit of one no-carb day each week, the weight should fall away.

Like any weight-loss diet, adopting the Honey Diet will mean making a few adjustments to when and how you eat, but I have made things as simple as possible by detailing a meal-by-meal plan below. Follow this plan on six days of the week, then turn to page 85 for an example of how to eat on your one no-carb day.

But before you start, check out the Honey Diet shopping list on page 84 and stock up your kitchen with delicious, healthy food.

THE HONEY DIET DAY (PHASE 2)

Forget about picking, nibbling and grazing your way through the day, the Honey Diet requires you to commit to eating four regular meals a day – breakfast, lunch and dinner and, VERY importantly (absolutely crucial), your 'fifth meal' of 1 to 2 tablespoons (50g) of honey just before you go to bed.

AS SOON AS YOU WAKE UP

Instead of reaching for a cup of coffee or tea, get into the habit of starting your day with a honey drink before breakfast (1 to 2 teaspoons of honey in hot water with a squeeze of lemon juice). This is all it takes to 'prime' your liver after the 8-hour night-time fast, relax your brain and calm any stress hormones that might be swimming around your system. That early morning cup of tea or coffee on an empty stomach might be what it usually takes to get you out of bed, but that's because it triggers a spike in adrenaline which could be enough to get your harmful, unwanted stress hormones on the move.

BREAKFAST

If you like cereal in the morning, be careful, as most are VERY high in sugar, which can trigger cravings for the rest of the day. Even an apparently 'healthy' variety like bran flakes contains up to 4 teaspoons of sugar per bowl, before you even think about sprinkling extra on top!

Opt for no-added-sugar muesli, Weetabix (drizzle with honey not sugar), Shredded Wheat (add a little honey or frozen berries) or porridge made with half water, half milk and a little honey, to taste.

Try to include some form of protein (either eggs or grilled bacon or cheese or ham) with your breakfast when you can because studies show it keeps hunger hormones at bay and will ensure you eat less during the rest of the day.

Try one slice of wholemeal/multi-grain bread with:

● 2 eggs (poached, boiled or scrambled)
● 2 grilled rashers of bacon and a grilled tomato

Or, for breakfast on the move, sandwich two rice cakes together with a generous slice of Brie and ham.

● Plain yoghurt (2 to 3 tablespoons) with honey and fruit (from your 2-piece allowance)

Plus tea or coffee (sweetened with honey if desired, not sugar)

LUNCH

Try soup, ideally one with lentils/beans/meat/fish (to provide protein), plus two oatcakes and a slice of cheese, if you're hungry.

Alternatively, make a pot of salad to take to work with you – just ensure it contains some form of protein such as tinned tuna, a boiled egg, ham or cold chicken.

If you didn't have toast or cereal for breakfast, enjoy a sandwich with wholemeal bread and a protein-based filling such as salami and sun-dried tomatoes, pâté and mixed peppers, tuna, cheese or ham (aim for an open sandwich, with more filling than bread if possible).

If you had an egg-free breakfast, make yourself an omelette/egg on toast.

If you are hungry mid-morning or mid-afternoon, choose from:

- 2 oatcakes with a thin slice of cheese, hummus or almond butter
- Piece of fruit (to a maximum of 2 per day)
- Small handful of nuts/seeds/dried fruit (dates/sultanas/raisins/apricots)
- 2 to 3 wholegrain breadsticks with hummus
- Wholewheat crackers, oatcakes or rice cakes spread with peanut butter
- A few cherry tomatoes
- Crudités of cucumber, celery and carrot

DINNER (7 TO 9PM – EAT AS LATE AS POSSIBLE)

If this is your main meal, it should be predominantly made up of vegetables or salad (with an olive oil-based dressing) with a palm-sized piece of grilled or steamed protein (fish, lean meat) and a fist-sized portion of wholegrain carbohydrates.

The important issue is to ensure you are getting a portion of protein with every meal and to keep carbohydrates WHOLEMEAL and in smaller quantities than you are probably used to. Try to steer clear of pasta meals, risotto and special fried rice. Instead, discover a wealth of options based on meat/fish and vegetables.

It is worth scouring the shelves of health food shops for grains like quinoa, which looks and tastes a bit like brown rice but is high in protein and low in carbohydrate.

As long as the meal contains a palm-sized portion of protein, and plenty of different salads or vegetables, you will be on message for the Honey Diet. Just keep carbohydrate portions small.

Try:

- Mince with onions, peppers, courgettes and tomatoes, seasoned with oregano and served with a small portion of wholewheat pasta or topped with sweet potato and a grating of strongly flavoured cheese
- Liver and bacon with onion gravy and cauliflower
- Ham and cheese omelette with a side salad
- Smoked mackerel with a mixed salad and ready-cooked beetroot
- Pork casserole with beans and tomatoes
- Beef stir-fry with a small portion of brown rice or wholewheat noodles
- Chicken curry with apples, apricots, sultanas, tomatoes and coconut milk served with a small portion of brown rice

- Cauliflower cheese with peas and cherry tomatoes
- Meatballs in tomato sauce with a small portion of wholewheat pasta

If you have a sweet tooth, you can finish your meal with a dessertspoon of berries or fruits, topped with any of the following:

- Yoghurt
- Sour cream or crème fraîche
- Chopped nuts
- Shredded coconut

Or a small pot of yoghurt with honey.

Alternatively, try oatcakes or rice cakes with a small piece (matchbox-sized) of cheese.

BEDTIME

1 to 2 tablespoons of honey within 30 minutes of going to bed.

Take the honey in hot water (possibly with a dash of fruit juice or a squeeze of lemon to add flavour), herbal tea, spread on crispbread or stirred into plain yoghurt.

Aim for 8 hours' sleep.

OLIVE OIL

Use olive oil as your principal fat in salad dressings or 'dry fry' in a pan rubbed with a few drops of olive oil or a squirt of olive oil spray. Although fat in the diet isn't as bad for you as sugar, it helps to keep calorie intake down when trying to lose weight. Furthermore, olive oil contains oleic acids, a type of monounsaturated fat, which help control bad (LDL) cholesterol levels while raising good (HDL) cholesterol. The fats in olives also boost levels of serotonin, the feel-good brain chemical.

NUTS

If you get hungry between meals, it's a good idea to snack on nuts – up to a small handful of, ideally unsalted, nuts (such as almonds, cashews and walnuts) each day. Most nuts contain unsaturated fats, which are good for heart health. They are also rich in the antioxidant vitamin E, folic acid (which reduces levels of the dangerous amino acid homocysteine in the blood) and plant fibre (which can reduce cholesterol levels). In addition, nuts contain arginine, which is a precursor to nitric acid, a substance made in the walls of blood vessels that relaxes the blood vessels and prevents clotting.

Studies have shown that 3 to 4 tablespoons of nuts, five times a week, can reduce the incidence of coronary disease by 25 to 39 per cent.

TIME FOR A DRINK?

Studies show that people who drink alcohol moderately are a little healthier than those who don't drink at all and moderate amounts of alcohol have been shown to increase the level of good cholesterol in the blood.

If you're going to drink, red wine is possibly best. It contains the antioxidant resveratrol, which may provide some protection against heart disease, and scientists believe the salicylates in red wine (which come from the grape skin) interfere with the processes that lead to cancer, heart disease and even Alzheimer's. Some studies have suggested that the chemical phenylethylamine in red wine triggers the release of dopamine, a feel-good brain chemical.

Try to stick to one (small) glass a day with your evening meal, but avoid if you have quite a bit of weight to lose, and avoid drinking in excess. More than 2 units per day puts you at risk of health problems, including cancer. It will affect your sleep, too, and reduce the efficiency of your nocturnal fat burning.

SHOPPING LIST

If you are committed to losing weight with the Honey Diet, it is worth doing a little bit of preparatory groundwork before you start. Scour your kitchen cupboards and fridge for anything in a packet, scrutinize those labels and clear out everything containing sugar or sweeteners in their many forms (glucose, fructose, corn syrup, dextrose, lactose, maltodextrin, maltose, sucrose, xylose, aspartame, saccharin, sucralose etc), anything made from white flour (bread, biscuits, crackers) along with any processed or convenience foods (ready meals etc). This diet is based on simple, natural wholefoods, so stock up instead on:

HONEY

LEAN MEAT (chicken, turkey, beef, bacon, lamb, pork, ham, veal and high-meat content hamburgers and sausages)

EGGS

FISH (all types – fresh, tinned or frozen, but not in breadcrumbs or batter)

SALADS (avocado, cucumber, lettuce, radishes, spring onions, sprouts – bean and alfalfa, tomato, watercress)

VEGETABLES (artichoke, asparagus, beetroot, broccoli, Brussels sprouts, cauliflower, cabbage, celery, courgette, green beans, kale, leek, mushrooms, onion, pepper, pumpkin, rhubarb, shallots, spinach, squash, turnip)

PULSES (beans, lentils)

FRUIT – especially berries (frozen is fine)

OLIVE OIL SPRAY

HERBS/SPICES/SEASONING

FULL-FAT DAIRY PRODUCTS (plain bio-yoghurt, cottage cheese, all forms of cheese, milk – although semi-skimmed is fine if you prefer)

STORE CUPBOARD wholemeal flour (plain and self-raising for baking), wholewheat pasta/noodles, brown rice, no-sugar cereals, oats, dried fruit, nuts, oatcakes, rice cakes, ryvita, no-sugar peanut butter

YOUR NO-CARB DAY

Once you get into the swing of it, it's easy to get through one day without carbohydrates – there's no need to feel hungry!

Wake up to a cup of hot water with honey and a squeeze of lemon.

BREAKFAST OPTIONS

- 2 grilled rashers of bacon and a grilled tomato
- 2 small sausages and an apple
- Kippers
- 2 slices of cold ham and salad
- Grilled bacon and fried eggs with mushrooms

LUNCH OPTIONS

- Soup
- Salad with some form of protein (eggs, ham, tuna, cheese) or make your own healthy combination of tuna with mashed butter beans and mayonnaise or a three-bean salad mixed with Stilton or sliced avocado and prawns with basil and tomato
- Omelette with ham/mushrooms/tomatoes/cheese

DINNER OPTIONS

- A palm-sized portion of meat or fish of any kind with as much salad or vegetables as you like. Try any of the meal suggestions on on pages 81–2, but just avoid the pasta, rice, potatoes or bread with your evening meal today
- In place of ordinary carbs, look out for no-carb noodles and pasta (made from yam)
- Finish your meal with yoghurt sprinkled with seeds and honey or a piece of cheese – avoid fruit today

OPTIONAL SNACKS

- Handful of nuts
- Crudités dipped into hummus
- Cream cheese whipped up with tiny pieces of smoked salmon

Late-night honey drink

Chapter 6

USING HONEY IN YOUR COOKING

SWITCH TO HONEY STRAIGHTAWAY

Use honey as a:

- Drizzle for desserts – on fruit, in yoghurt, on cereals
- Sweetener for tea, coffee or smoothies
- Seasoning for barbecue spare ribs, pork chops or chicken wings before cooking
- Salad dressing with olive oil and vinegar

BAKING WITH HONEY

1. Honey is twice as sweet as sugar, so, when substituting in baking, halve the sugar quantity for honey. Because honey is hygroscopic (meaning it attracts water), you also need to reduce the amount of liquid in the recipe by 50ml for 250ml of honey added.

2. When baking with honey, beat your mixture more vigorously and for longer than you would when adding sugar.

3. Add ½ teaspoon bicarbonate of soda for each cup of honey used in place of sugar in baking. This will neutralize honey's acidity and help the mixture rise.
4. Reduce the oven temperature very slightly as honey makes the mixture crisper and brown faster than a sugar one.

MEASURING HONEY ACCURATELY

Smear, spray or brush the inside walls of your measuring cup or spoons with a thin layer of oil before pouring out the required amount of honey. This prevents the honey from sticking on to the cup.

RECIPES

SPECIAL PORRIDGE

This delicious morning porridge is adapted from one created by Allegra McEvedy.

Serves 1
2 heaped tbsp porridge oats
1 tsp sultanas
250ml water or semi-skimmed milk
2 dried apricots or almonds, chopped
1 tsp honey

Put the oats, sultanas and water or milk in a non-stick pan and simmer for 10 minutes, stirring frequently. Pour into a bowl, scatter the apricots or almonds on top and drizzle over the honey.

CLASSIC MUESLI

A Bircher-style muesli that is a great summer alternative to porridge, created by Allegra McEvedy.

Serves 1
1 heaped tbsp rolled oats
2 dried apricots, chopped
2 tbsp unsweetened apple juice
½ apple
1 tbsp natural yoghurt
3 brazil nuts, chopped
1 tsp clear honey

The evening before, put the oats, chopped apricots and apple juice in a bowl, stir, cover and leave overnight. The following morning, grate in the unpeeled apple, add the yoghurt and stir. Toast the chopped nuts in a frying pan until they begin to colour and scatter over the muesli. Drizzle with the honey.

HONEY GRANOLA

This crunchy cereal uses honey instead of sugar and is much cheaper (and tastier!) than shop-bought.

Makes 1kg
250g rolled oats
100g wheat bran
150g sunflower seeds
150g honey
60ml groundnut oil
100g hazelnuts
150g dates

100g dried apricots
100g wheatgerm
100g sultanas

Preheat the oven to 180°C (gas mark 4). Mix the rolled oats, wheat bran and sunflower seeds together in a large bowl. Heat the honey in a pan with the oil until the honey has melted. Pour over the dry mix. Stir well and spread over a large baking tray. Roast for 20 minutes, turning three to four times. Meanwhile, roast the hazelnuts in the same oven for about 10 minutes, then roughly chop them with the dates and dried apricots. When the granola is cool, stir in the nuts and fruit, the wheatgerm and sultanas.

HONEY ENERGY BARS

A delicious snack based on Hugh Fearnley-Whittingstall's honey and peanut butter booster bars. The bars are fuelled with honey, not sugar, and will keep for 5 to 7 days in an airtight tin.

Makes 16
125g unsalted butter
125g crunchy peanut butter
150g honey, plus extra to drizzle
Finely grated zest of 1 orange
Finely grated zest of 1 lemon
200g porridge oats
150g dried fruit (raisins, sultanas, chopped apricots, prunes, dates)
150g mixed seeds

Preheat the oven to 160°C (gas mark 3). Grease and line a baking tin, about 20cm square. Put the butter, peanut butter, honey and grated citrus zests in a deep saucepan over a very low heat. Leave until melted, stirring occasionally. Pour in the oats, dried fruit and three-quarters of the seeds and stir until combined. Spread evenly in the baking tin and smooth the top. Scatter the remaining seeds over the surface and trickle with a little more honey. Bake for about 30 minutes, until golden in the centre and golden brown at the edges. Leave to cool completely in the tin, then turn out and cut into squares with a sharp knife.

FRUITY HONEY SMOOTHIE

This tasty smoothie is loaded with bioflavonoids. (Thanks to www.benefits-of-honey.com.)

Serves 1
½ banana
5 strawberries
250g plain yoghurt
2 tsp honey
Ice cubes

Cut up the banana into pieces and put them into a blender with the strawberries. Add the yoghurt, honey and ice cubes. Blend the mixture to make a delicious, smooth, cool drink.

CINNAMON HONEY BUTTER

Another recipe from www.benefits-of-honey.com. This makes a delicious sweet breakfast spread.

Makes 250g
60g soft butter
¼ tsp ground cinnamon
175g honey
1 tbsp cream cheese (optional)

Blend all the ingredients together in a bowl and beat well until the mixture is smooth and creamy. Spread the butter on piping hot toast or wholemeal crackers.

HONEY CAKE

The idea for this lovely nutty honey cake came from *The Kitchen Revolution* by Rosie Sykes, Polly Russell and Zoe Heron.

Makes 1 x 20cm cake
1 lemon
150ml milk
5 eggs
½ tsp baking powder
125g semolina
125g ground almonds
7 tbsp clear honey
A pinch of salt
Butter, for greasing

Preheat the oven to 180°C (gas mark 4) and lightly grease a 20cm by 10cm deep cake tin. Grate the zest of the lemon and squeeze out its juice, adding the juice to the milk. Separate the eggs and sift the baking powder into a bowl with the semolina and almonds. Whisk the egg yolks with the lemon zest and honey until light and fluffy. Separately, whisk the egg whites with a pinch of salt until they form soft peaks. Stir the baking powder, semolina and almonds into the yolk mixture, add the milk and blend until smooth. Gradually fold in the egg whites and pour into the cake tin. Bake for 40 minutes or until the cake is firm. Slice while still warm and serve with Greek yoghurt and honey.

HONEY BANANA MUFFINS

A healthier version of muffins using a small amount of honey instead of spoons of table sugar. (From www.benefits-of-honey.com.) Add 2 tablespoons cocoa powder to the flour for a chocolate version.

Makes 10–12

3 big bananas, mashed

5 tbsp honey

1 egg

2 tbsp melted butter

75ml sunflower oil

225g wholemeal flour

1 tsp baking powder

1 tsp bicarbonate of soda

½ tsp salt

For the banana cinnamon crumble topping

1 small banana, sliced

2 tbsp plain flour

½ tsp ground cinnamon

1 tsp set honey

1 tbsp frozen butter

Preheat the oven to 190°C (gas mark 5) and line a 12-cup muffin tin with paper muffin cases. Beat the bananas, honey, egg, melted butter and oil together for a few minutes in a bowl. Mix together the flour, baking powder, bicarbonate of soda and salt. Pour the banana mixture into the flour mixture and blend well. Spoon the batter into the muffin cases. Place one banana slice on top of each muffin. To make the crumble topping, mix the flour, cinnamon and honey in a bowl. Rub in the butter and sprinkle the topping over the muffins. Bake for 20 minutes until a toothpick inserted into the muffins comes out clean.

CHEWY HONEY PRETZELS

Soft pretzels with honey and cinnamon are irresistible. (Recipe from www.benefits-of-honey.com.)

Makes about 12
1 tsp dry yeast
4 tbsp honey
A pinch of sea salt
225g wholemeal flour
150g wholemeal bread flour
2 tbsp bicarbonate of soda
4 tbsp melted butter
1 tbsp ground cinnamon

Dissolve the dry yeast, 2 tablespoons of the honey and a pinch of sea salt in 250ml warm water. Add to the two flours in a mixing bowl and bring together to form a dough. Knead the dough on a lightly floured surface until smooth and elastic. This is a critical step to achieve that soft and chewy texture for the pretzels. Leave to rise for 45 minutes. When the dough has doubled its size, pinch off bits and roll into long ropes 1cm thin. Leave in a warm place to rise for about half an hour. Preheat the oven to 220°C (gas mark 7). Roll the dough once more into really thin ropes and shape as desired. Make a soda bath by mixing 500ml warm water with the bicarbonate of soda. Stir well, then dip the pretzels into it. Place the dipped pretzels on a well-greased baking tray. Bake the pretzels for about 10 minutes until golden brown. Make a honey butter mixture by blending the melted butter with the remaining honey and brush over the warm pretzels. Sprinkle the ground cinnamon over the top and serve warm.

SOFT MOIST BANANA CAKE

This cake is spongy, soft, moist and bursting with the irresistible fragrance of fresh bananas! (Recipe from www.benefits-of-honey. com.)

Makes 1 x 23cm cake
3 eggs, at room temperature
6 tbsp honey
6 very ripe small bananas or 3 big bananas
180g wholemeal self-raising flour
½ tsp baking powder
¼ tsp bicarbonate of soda
80ml sunflower oil
2 tbsp melted butter

Preheat the oven to 170°C (gas mark 3–4) and grease and flour the bottom of a 23cm cake tin (do not grease the sides). Whisk the eggs at maximum speed until stiff, then add the honey and whisk until it doubles in volume. Mash the bananas and add them to the mixture, mixing everything together with a spatula. Sift in the flour, baking powder and bicarbonate of soda and gently fold in. Do not over-fold the batter. Mix about a third of the batter with the oil and butter and blend well. Pour the oil mixture into the rest of the batter and gently mix well. Pour the batter into the prepared tin and bake the cake for 40–45 minutes on the lower rack of the oven (this helps the cake rise better). The cake is ready when it is golden brown and a skewer inserted into the cake comes out clean. Before removing the cake, invert the tin on to a rack and leave until completely cool to give the cake a nice height.

HONEY ROLLS

These honey rolls are sweeter than normal bread rolls and so are delicious for tea. Recipe from www.benefits-of-honey.com.

Serves 5–6

For the dough
50g wholemeal flour
220g plain flour
2 tsp dry yeast
2 tsp milk powder
1 tsp sea salt
1 tbsp honey
30g melted butter
½ egg, beaten
125ml water

For the glaze
½ egg (the remaining half!)
1 tbsp milk

60g raisins (optional)

Mix all the ingredients for the dough in a big bowl and stir to form a dough. Spread some bread flour on the table to prevent the dough from sticking and knead it with your fingers for about 10 minutes. Gather and fold the ends of the dough towards you and push it away, repeating the action again and again until the dough's texture becomes soft and smooth. The dough should spring back when lightly pressed with a finger. Set aside in a warm place for 30–40 minutes, to allow the dough to double in size, then flatten the dough with your hands. Preheat the oven to 180°C (gas mark 4). If you want to, add raisins on the flattened dough, then fold and roll it up. Cut the roll into small equal sections and shape each one into an oval with the palm of your hand. Grease a baking tray with olive oil. Rest all the pieces on the tray for another 30–40 minutes to allow a second rising. The pieces should become twice as big. Slash the middle of each roll with a knife. Make the glaze by mixing together the egg and milk, then brush a layer of the glazing mixture over the top of each roll. Bake in the oven for about 15–20 minutes until golden. Serve either hot or cool with butter or cinnamon honey butter spread (see page 91).

CHOCOLATE CHIP HONEY ROLLS

If it seems too much effort to weigh everything out, try this simple recipe using measuring cups. Just follow the method for the www.benefits-of-honey.com rolls above.

Serves 5–6

For the dough
2 cups wholemeal bread flour
2 tsp dry yeast
2 tsp milk powder
1 tsp sea salt
1 tbsp honey
2 tbsp melted butter
½ egg, beaten
½ cup water

For the glaze
½ egg (the remaining half!)
1 tbsp milk
½–¾ cup (or as much as you like) choc chips

Use the same method as above, adding the choc chips to the dough in the same way you added the raisins, if using.

RAISIN HONEY BREAD

You can use the breadmaking method from the last two recipes to turn your rolls into a delicious loaf, perfect for toasting. This recipe is from www.benefits-of-honey.com and also has some nutritious oat bran added to it.

Makes 1 loaf
50g oat bran
220g wholemeal bread flour
2 tsp instant dry yeast
2 tsp milk powder
1 tsp sea salt
1 tbsp honey
30g melted butter
½ egg, beaten
125ml water

For the glaze
½ egg (the remaining half!)
1 tbsp milk

60g raisins or dried cranberries
50g muesli flakes or sesame seeds

Use the same method as for the honey rolls to make the dough, adding the raisins or cranberries to the dough after the first rising, but not cutting the roll up. Grease a loaf tin with olive oil. Rest the dough in the tin for another 30–40 minutes to allow a second rising. The dough should become twice as big. Make the glaze by mixing together the egg and milk, then brush a layer of the glazing mixture over the top of the dough in the tin. Sprinkle the muesli flakes or sesame seeds on top to make the crust even crunchier.

Bake in the oven for about 20 minutes until the top of the loaf is golden. Serve either hot or cool with butter or cinnamon honey butter spread (see page 91).

APPLE AND WALNUT COOKIES

Packed with nutrients, these cookies from Louise Atkinson make a great snack.

Makes 12–15
75g wholemeal flour
75g rolled oats
½ tsp baking powder
½ tsp ground cinnamon
1 apple, peeled, cored and grated
50g walnuts, chopped
75g honey
60ml sunflower oil
Zest of ½ orange

Preheat the oven to 180°C (gas mark 4). Stir the flour, oats, baking powder and cinnamon together in a bowl. Add the apple and nuts and stir again. In a separate bowl, mix together the honey, oil and orange zest. Combine the wet and dry ingredients. Place heaped tablespoons of the mixture on to a lined baking tray, leaving a 5cm space between each one, and bake for 10 minutes.

RHUBARB AND BANANA CRUNCHY CRUMBLE

A delightful sugar-free pudding based on a recipe from *The Balance Diet* by Jennifer Irvine.

Serves 2

For the filling
200g rhubarb, cut into 1cm chunks
Juice of 1 orange
1 tbsp honey

For the topping
25ml sunflower oil
2 tbsp honey
30g ground almonds
50g porridge oats
Zest of ½ orange
½ teaspoon ground cinnamon
A handful of pecans, roughly chopped (optional)
1 ripe banana, sliced

Preheat the oven to 180°C (gas mark 4). Bring the rhubarb, orange juice and 1 tablespoon of the honey slowly to the boil in a non-stick saucepan. Reduce the heat, cover and allow to simmer for 5 minutes until the rhubarb is soft. To make the topping, in a mixing bowl combine the oil and honey, then add the almonds, oats, orange zest, cinnamon and pecans and stir to cover everything. Pour the rhubarb into a small ovenproof dish and top with slices of banana, then scatter over the crumble mixture. Cook the crumble for 15–20 minutes until the top is browned and the fruit bubbling.

Chapter 7

BOOST YOUR BRAIN POWER

The Honey Diet isn't just about weight control, it will fuel your brain, improve your memory and concentration, and protect you against the ravages of mental ageing.

Have you ever walked into a room and then wondered what on earth you were doing there? Do you sometimes have trouble remembering names? Or where you might have left the car keys? Or what you got up to yesterday or last weekend?

You can blame your age, a hectic lifestyle, having too much on your plate, but the tricky truth is your brain is probably shrinking.

We all experience a degree of brain shrinkage as we get older, as the cells die and are not replaced, and our oh-so-important grey matter shrinks at a rate of around 1 per cent per year after middle age. There's not much we can do about that.

But if we allow our brain to get hungry – either because we eat too much sugar and junk food, or we don't get enough sleep – our brain will release a cascade of stress hormones, which studies show put it at risk of accelerated shrinkage.

The same hungry brain reactions that are making us fat, and ruining our sleep, are also shrinking our very delicate brains.

It's frightening, but if you follow the Honey Diet you can reverse the whole process – making you sharper and better able to concentrate, and improving your memory.

THE iPUMP AND IQ

If you ask most specialists about the possible causes of dementia and Alzheimer's, they will typically blame furring of the tiny blood vessels of the brain, which, they believe, restricts blood supply, resulting in neurones in whole areas of the brain being starved out of action. But I believe the problem is triggered by a short-circuiting of the tiny iPump in each glial cell.

Studies show that obese children who live on a high-sugar junk food diet (and who would be expected to have iPumps on permanent switch-off) are more likely to have a lower IQ than normal-weight children. They are so young that their obesity, even if it triggered diabetes, couldn't possibly have had time to block the tiny blood vessels in the brain as it might in older obese adults. I believe they are suffering symptoms of a hungry brain.

The stress signals sent out by a hungry brain also explain the excitability and hyperactivity in children so often associated with high-sugar diets. It is not the sugar causing the reaction, it is the stress response of the hungry brain, which happens because the sugar has tripped the child's iPump yet again.

BRAIN HUNGER CAUSES BOTH WEIGHT GAIN AND DEMENTIA

I think it is pretty sinister to think that just as obesity levels have steadily risen over recent years, so have recorded incidences of memory loss, dementias and Alzheimer's disease.

Our physical and mental health parameters are declining in tandem, and with increasing acceleration. Rates of weight gain, diabetes and Alzheimer's disease are doubling every two decades. Statistics show that the steady rise in obesity and diabetes since the 1970s correlates alarmingly with a gradual fall in IQ.

There are currently 35 million sufferers of Alzheimer's disease around the world, and even conservative estimates suggest that within 100 years the number of Alzheimer's patients will top 1 billion, obesity several billions.

I am convinced that this is no coincidence. Brain hunger is the key. It is causing BOTH weight gain and dementia.

The modern high-sugar junk food diet means we are all eating far too much sugar and this is tripping the iPump, dramatically reducing the fuel supply to the brain.

Without sufficient fuel for any length of time, the brain cells begin to wither and die.

Brain scans show that people with dementia have damaged brain cells, and the pattern of damage follows a path of accelerated ageing. Normally, as we age, learned memories will be the first to be knocked out (or at least sacrificed) as the brain shuts down the very fuel-hungry memory regions of the brain that our hunter/gatherer ancestors would not necessarily have needed beyond a certain age.

Basic motor functions (such as walking, feeding, washing) that you need to live are usually left intact.

It is no coincidence that diseases like dementia and Alzheimer's specifically target the memory and learning regions of the brain, too. Even with advanced Alzheimer's, a patient would still be able to walk and dress themselves (the brain signals to their arms and legs remaining unscathed) until the point where they lose the memory for the correct sequence of actions – and stand looking at their clothes, wondering what they are supposed to do with them.

You might notice a certain foggy-headedness or occasional difficulties in concentration as you get older, but if you have been eating a high-sugar diet likely to trip your iPump on a regular basis, it could be that your brain cells are not getting a regular and efficient fuel supply. They might be dying off much faster than they should.

A hungry brain doesn't just shut down quietly. It will typically trigger a massive stress response throughout the body in its quest for more fuel, and I am convinced that this makes things worse.

The stress hormone cortisol, for instance, is known to damage brain tissue. Studies of post-traumatic stress victims show that a prolonged burst of cortisol (released as a result of intense stress) can be powerful enough to shrink the brain's memory stores.

If your brain is stressed because it is hungry, you could be knocking out potentially useful brain function far earlier in life than you need to. You could even be putting yourself at increased risk of dementia and Alzheimer's.

Autopsies of people with modern neurological diseases such as motor neurone disease and Parkinson's have shown that many of their problems are driven by loss of function of glial cells. These are the 'feeder' cells for the neurones, which house the iPumps.

Although they don't do the actual thinking, the glial cells are known to be extremely important. In fact, they are key to all human information processing – to vision, consciousness, cognition, thought and language. When brain experts want to measure the development of higher functions in animals (and humans), they count the number of glial cells they can find.

For instance, autopsies of Einstein's brain found it to be no bigger than anyone else's brain, but it had a greater number of those iPump-housing glial cells than most people. His brain was clearly highly efficient at pumping in fuel.

I am convinced that Alzheimer's is not so much a disease as a physiological adaptation to a low energy supply to the brain cells caused by tripped iPumps.

But you might just be able to protect yourself from the damage that leads to these hideously debilitating conditions if you adapt your diet in such a way as to ensure your iPump functions day and night as it should. By adopting the principles of the Honey Diet, you will be doing the best you can to protect your iPump and ensure a steady fuel supply to your brain, so that it can remain active, sharp, vibrant and alive for as long as possible.

IMPROVING YOUR CREATIVE THINKING

The quiet moments between meetings or between highly focussed mental or physical tasks are incredibly important for the brain. You might think you've switched off and you're in a kind of 'mental neutral gear', but this is when the brain cells are freed from a particular energy-demanding task and can engage in offline unconscious creative thinking.

These are the moments when the energy demands of the brain (during the day) are at their highest. It might appear to have powered down, but actually the brain has powered up, and is doing the work for us unconsciously without troubling our conscious minds.

This explains how, when you are completely foxed by a conundrum, if you take a short break – walk away, do something else – the answer might pop into your head, even though you weren't consciously thinking about it at the time.

But this will only work if your brain has a ready supply of fuel, your iPump is working as it should, and your liver's glycogen stores are well stocked.

That's what the Honey Diet will do.

SUGAR ADDICTION

Sugar has a complex and important relationship with the brain. There is no doubt that it is a highly addictive substance.

If a drug addict is deprived of their fix for a few hours they may feel bad, but they are unlikely to die from withdrawal. If the human brain is deprived of sugar for a few minutes, it begins to die as neurones gradually shut down. If you deny it its fix, the only way the brain can cope is to instigate a coma, where all non-vital processes are locked down and all systems are mobilized to defend the brain's energy supply. No other addictive substance or drug causes such a catastrophic meltdown if withdrawn for a few minutes.

Without its sugar 'fix', the brain is only ever minutes away from coma.

Just like a junkie or an alcoholic, the more sugar we have, the more we want. When the palate is dulled by overconsumption, we need even more sugar to get the same 'high'.

But honey is a very different kind of sugar. It is the only food that can fix this destructive cycle.

Chapter 8

PROTECT YOURSELF AGAINST AGEING AND DISEASE

You will know by now that the Honey Diet will, as well as helping you lose weight, also improve your sleep, help you burn fat throughout the night, boost your brain power and protect you from memory loss and dementia. However, perhaps the most stunning additional benefit of adopting the Honey Diet is the fact that this new way of eating could go a long way to protecting you against the slide into old age.

Diseases like diabetes and heart disease and osteoporosis, depression, infertility and poor immunity are taking younger and younger victims all the time, with their incidence reaching epidemic proportions. Many experts now believe that the modern diet of sugar and junk food has a lot to answer for.

Over the years, there have been hundreds of thousands of studies trying to reach an understanding of this apparent acceleration of diseases that occur naturally as part of the ageing process, and in many cases the finger of blame has pointed to stress.

There is no doubt that stress hormones like cortisol and adrenaline have a highly corrosive effect on our bodies, and play a very important part in the toxic overload that exacerbates our tendency to age: from wrinkles to heart disease.

Many scientists blame our stressful modern lifestyles and ponder the possibility that we have not evolved sufficiently well to cope with the pressures of the computer age, 24-hour media and unlimited choice, etc.

But I believe that psychosocial stress pales into insignificance when compared to the catastrophic whole-body impact of the constant, all-pervading stress of the hungry brain.

Most of us are awash with stress hormones not because of money worries, or marital concerns, but because our brains are always hungry.

If you are overweight or you, like the vast majority of the Western population, spend much of your day drinking fizzy drinks and nibbling at crisps, chips, cakes, biscuits, white buttered toast and pasta, there is every chance your iPump will be on permanent switch-off.

After just 15 minutes on emergency fuel rations when the iPump is off, the brain will start to get hungry.

A hungry brain is a stressed brain, sending out all sorts of toxic stress messages in its attempt to get more fuel. Some stress signals stimulate appetite, driving impossible-to-resist cravings, while others call up emergency stores of glucose from the liver, and more still instruct a process by which muscles are broken down to be converted to useful fuel.

These signals are very efficient and effectively raise blood sugar levels once more. However, the new levels of excess glucose swimming around in the blood trigger the release of a massive rise in insulin, which carries the glucose off to be stored as fat (not a good thing).

The wave of new glucose that does reach the glial cells is very often so intense it ensures the iPump STAYS switched off. So the brain remains hungry and continues to pump out stress hormones.

The real worry is the fact that the brain's stress hormones can be very toxic to the body.

The main stress hormone, cortisol, appears to have a side effect whereby it inadvertently dulls the cells' response to insulin. This can make us increasingly 'insulin resistant', encouraging the body to pump out more and more insulin in its efforts to get some sort of response. Other stress hormones, such as adrenaline, speed up the heart and tighten the arteries, raising blood pressure.

It is these hormones, and this insulin overload, that REALLY increase our risk of degenerating diseases.

Whether this effect manifests itself as osteoporosis, obesity, heart disease or wrinkles will depend, to some extent, on your genetic profile and your natural 'tolerance' of junk food and sugar.

Some of us will eventually become diabetic, some obese, some will have heart problems, others will become demented or succumb to full-blown Alzheimer's disease. Our genes play a large part, but so do lifestyle factors. It is clear to me that one of the worst things you can do – apart from smoking – is fill your belly with high-energy sugary and processed foods.

The bitter truth is that if we carry on eating badly, most of us will succumb in some way to something horrible as a consequence of the energy overload in the modern diet.

The Honey Diet is the first step in reversing this process. It is carefully calculated to ensure that the brain is adequately fuelled – day and night – and therefore has no need to pump out destructive stress hormones.

So by adopting the Honey Diet, you won't just be losing weight, you will be reducing your risk of a very frightening array of degenerative diseases.

HEART DISEASE

We are all conditioned to believe that heart disease is exacerbated by dietary fat – specifically saturated fat – and there is no doubt that fats in the blood do cling to artery walls, narrowing and hardening them. But studies show this only happens as a result of the action of stress hormones.

For decades we have been blaming the alarming rise in heart disease statistics on dietary fat and 'executive stress'. I am convinced that the culprit is not so much executive stress as metabolic stress triggered by a hungry brain.

Here's how it works: the stress hormone adrenaline speeds up the heart and tightens the arteries, raising blood pressure. As part of the stress response, the clotting ability of the blood increases (your blood thickens to prepare your body in the event of injury). Together, these two factors increase your risk of heart attack and stroke.

At the same time, the stress hormone cortisol triggers insulin resistance. Insulin is supposed to help with the transport system by which glucose (fuel) gets into the cells that line the stomach. But because of the action of cortisol, the cells that line our arteries become resistant to the insulin and don't get the glucose that they need. The arterial cells soon become hungry and can begin to malfunction. As the blood vessel walls start to break down, they increasingly attract fat molecules swimming around in the blood. Because the walls are damaged, these lipids (blood fats) can very easily stick to the artery walls instead of passing through. This is atherosclerosis – the furring up of the arteries so common in heart disease.

This explains why people with diabetes have an increased risk of heart disease. Their long-term higher blood glucose levels increase the chance of damaged arteries, which means they are more likely to attract fat deposits to fur them up.

It is clear that blood fats wouldn't be clogging the arteries if it weren't for the damage to the arteries caused by stress. And in most cases today, this stress is caused by a high-sugar diet's impact on the brain.

This distinction also explains how some remote Arctic populations can live quite healthily on a diet made up predominantly of whale fat. That's about as saturated a fat as it is possible to have. But as long as the Inuits keep away from junk food (to keep glucose, and therefore insulin, levels low), their hearts stay healthy.

DIABETES

Type 1 diabetes occurs when the body suddenly stops producing insulin, but type 2 diabetes can occur when the cells THINK there is no insulin because they have become 'resistant' to it.

As I have explained before, the hungry brain chemical cascade (particularly the elevated levels of cortisol) can very swiftly lead to insulin resistance, which, if unchecked, can lead to type 2 diabetes. I am convinced the malfunctioning iPump and hungry brain is one very good reason why there are now nearly 3 million people in the UK with type 2 diabetes.

A switch to the Honey Diet is the best move you could possibly make to reverse your insulin resistance, and therefore your risk of diabetes.

Any diabetic will be warned off sugar, and honey will normally be included in the 'banned' list. However, as I explained in chapter 3, honey is actually extremely effective at stabilizing blood glucose levels (where ordinary sugar would do the opposite). Honey will also recalibrate the iPump. This means the Honey Diet is safe for people with type 2 diabetes.

Type 1 diabetes is more complex, so please consult your GP or specialist before making any dramatic changes to your diet.

GASTRIC PROBLEMS

The stress hormones pumped out by the hungry brain have a highly damaging effect on our digestive system. Quite simply, stress hormones cause your digestive system to shut down because your digestive system is the last thing you need to be worrying about if you are running away from a sabre-toothed tiger.

Shutting the gut down also helps protect the stomach lining from the corrosive effects of the stress hormone adrenaline. This is fine if the stress is short-lived, but if your brain is hungry and continually stressed, the hormones mean that your gut won't be functioning as it should and you will be getting little nutritional value from your food.

If you are stressed for long periods of time, the adrenaline can begin to degrade the extremely sensitive cells that line the gut, making you susceptible to food intolerances, gastric reflux problems and ulcers.

OSTEOPOROSIS

Long-term stress is extremely bad news for the health of your bones. Cortisol – even at not particularly high levels – can have a highly destructive effect on your bone density. It effectively breaks down bones because it interferes with the action of vitamin D in the digestive system, and in turn blocks the absorption of calcium (which should help make bones strong). Furthermore, less new bone is formed when there's cortisol around because the hormone stops the bone-building cells (the osteoblasts) from doing their job.

INFERTILITY

Anyone who has struggled to conceive will know that stress is no friend to conception. The problem is that cortisol can suppress normal functioning of the ovaries, which in turn leads to decreased production of the sex hormones that govern fertility. This is why women under extreme stress might notice that their periods stop temporarily.

Conception can be even more tricky, and menopause more likely, if you are insulin resistant. The condition can lead to disrupted ovulation for women and excessively high levels of androgens (male hormones).

POOR IMMUNITY

Poor immunity puts you at risk of every common cold or tummy bug going around, and can even increase your risk of cancer. Our immune strength will deplete naturally with age, but some people's immune system deteriorates faster than others. Stress is definitely BAD NEWS.

When the brain pumps out stress hormones, the immune system is temporarily closed down in an attempt to protect it from cortisol, which suppresses the immune system.

But if the stress is chronic (if you have long-term brain hunger), your immune system just won't be able to function efficiently – no matter how many vitamin C tablets you consume.

WRINKLES

We've all watched as people under extreme pressure (prime ministers and presidents, for instance) seem to age before our very eyes and it has long been suspected that stress accelerates the ageing process. What is clear is that prolonged stress (the sort a hungry brain might engender) means stress hormones are elevated for longer periods than they should, and our body can gradually wear down. The result is skin wrinkling, greying hair, painful joints, loss of hearing, declining sight – all the irritants people come to expect with age, but which, thanks to stress, come sooner.

One theory is that stress hormones cause chemical changes, which promote the visible signs of ageing we are so keen to delay.

Another is that stress and anxiety speed up the destruction of something called 'telomeres', which are the regions found at the ends of our chromosomes. Telomeres naturally diminish with age every time a cell divides and reproduces, but scientists believe stress speeds up the cell dying process, so resulting in muscle weakening, loss of eyesight and hearing, wrinkles and greying hair.

However, by switching to the Honey Diet you can immediately ensure your brain is well fed and not hungry. At night, this means the brain will be primed and in perfect condition to efficiently activate all the genes, hormones, enzymes and pathways that promote repair, recovery and restoration of all the tissues throughout the body while we sleep.

During the day, stress hormones will be minimized – or at least restricted to just making an appearance when we get stuck in a traffic jam or face a tricky deadline. The body can cope with occasional bursts of stress like this. It is the relentless onslaught triggered by the hungry brain that does so much damage.

We may not be able to avoid the stresses of modern life, but, by switching to the Honey Diet, we can avoid the destructive stress response of the hungry brain.

CONCLUSION

You may have picked up this book because you wanted to lose weight and, if so, you might have expected a draconian diet plan based on discomfort and hunger. But I really hope that by now you will have realized that if you eat the foods your body needs, it will work properly – both during the day and at night when you are asleep – and excess weight will fall off naturally.

I'd like to see a day when everyone who cares about their health follows phase 1 of the Honey Diet as a matter of course, and anyone who wants to lose a few pounds just dips into phase 2 until they achieve their target weight. Honey is such a powerful dietary tool that getting slim and staying there really should be as simple as that.

But the weight-loss aspect of the Honey Diet is merely the icing on the cake. Every day you spend following the Honey Diet is a day when your brain is not battling the vagaries of blood sugar peaks and troughs. It doesn't have to worry about being overloaded with sugar or about the possibility of a dwindling fuel supply.

While you follow the Honey Diet, your iPump will be working

just as it should, ensuring that a steady supply of nutrients reaches the neurones in your brain. If it's not hungry, your brain won't be stressed or shrinking. You will be able to think more clearly, be better able to concentrate and focus, and your memory will be pin sharp. Better still, you will be effectively protecting yourself against the ravages of dementia and Alzheimer's.

If your brain is Honey Diet happy, it won't be pumping stress hormones around your body, so your base-line stress levels will drop. This will instantly boost your immune system and reduce your risk of disease. From day one on the diet, you will sleep more soundly than you have ever slept before, and wake properly refreshed (both body and mind), having burnt up those pesky fat stores while you slept.

It is truly ridiculous how much good there is to be had from making such small dietary changes. You may merely be pleased that your jeans fit comfortably once more, and that your bulging waistline has disappeared, but, in truth, the long-term impact you are making on your health is far, far more significant than you ever thought possible.

And with something as delicious as honey, what's not to like? So please, enjoy honey in your diet, enjoy your new-found health and spread the word.

APPENDICES

APPENDIX A: THE SCIENCE BEHIND THE iPUMP

The key mechanisms of the glutamate/glutamine cycle (the iPump) were first articulated in 1999 by Magistretti and Pellerin at the Institute of Physiology, Faculty of Medicine in Lausanne, Switzerland, using brain imaging techniques.

They described the process as beginning with glutamate released from the neurone when it is low in ATP (fuel) which is then taken up by the astrocyte (glial cell). For each unit of glutamate taken up, one glucose molecule is pumped into the astrocyte:

'The stoichiometry of this process is such that for one glutamate molecule taken up with three Na+ ions, one glucose molecule enters an astrocyte, two ATP molecules are produced through aerobic glycolysis and two lactate molecules are released. Within the astrocyte, one ATP molecule fuels one "turn of the pump" while the other provides the energy needed to convert glutamate to glutamine by glutamine synthase. Evidence has been accumulated from structural as well as functional studies indicating that, under aerobic conditions, lactate may be the preferred energy substrate of activated neurons. Indeed, in the presence of oxygen, lactate is converted to pyruvate, which can be processed through the tricarboxylic acid cycle and the associated oxidative phosphorylation, to yield 17 ATP molecules per lactate molecule.'

At the cost of 2 molecules of ATP from glycolysis of glucose, 34 molecules (17 from each lactate molecule) are provided to the neurone for ongoing oxidative metabolism, to fund the energy of neurotransmission and all the numinous activities that we associate with being human – thought, language, cognition, tool making, social interaction, food sourcing, farming, civilization, writing, politics, law, learning, religion, literature, poetry, art and music.

This cycle is not exclusive to humans, but we are the only species that has developed a food culture that compromises this cycle.

APPENDIX B: HONEY AT NIGHT

Honey taken prior to sleep every night may constitute the single most significant and cost-effective contribution to public health and learning in several generations.

The mechanism by which honey improves sleep quality and recovery physiology is described by the HYMN (Honey/Insulin/Melatonin) Cycle. Each individual step of the cycle is well established and may be found in routine textbooks of biochemistry. The combined steps describe a cycle of metabolic activity that culminates in optimized recovery physiology during restorative sleep and, more importantly, in the reduction in the release of stress hormones during the night.

The cycle begins with the ingestion of 1 to 2 tablespoons of honey in the hour before bedtime and proceeds as follows:

1. The glucose portion of honey passes from the gut, through the liver circulation and into the general circulation, producing a mild glucose spike (glucose from honey produces only a mild or controlled elevation in blood sugar primarily because the fructose portion facilitates glucose uptake into the liver where it is converted to glycogen. Thus, less glucose reaches or remains in the general circulation.).
2. The mild elevation in blood sugar (from glucose) prompts a mild controlled release of insulin from the pancreas.
3. The presence of insulin in the general circulation drives tryptophan into the brain.
4. Tryptophan is converted to serotonin, a key hormone that promotes relaxation in the period prior to sleep.
5. In darkness, serotonin is converted to melatonin in the pineal gland – this is due to insulin promotion of noradrenaline, necessary to the conversion of serotonin to melatonin.
6. Melatonin activates sleep (by reducing body temperature and other mechanisms).
7. Melatonin also inhibits the release of more insulin from the pancreas, so preventing a rapid drop in blood sugar level.
8. Melatonin promotes the release of growth hormone by a circuitous route. The release of growth hormone (GH) is controlled by the activity of a growth-hormone-releasing hormone (GHRH). GHRH is in turn inhibited by another hormone – growth-hormone-releasing hormone inhibiting hormone. Melatonin inhibits this latter hormone, thus preventing the inhibition of GHRH, and therefore promoting the release of GH from the pituitary gland. GH is the hormone governing all of recovery physiology. This is the key first step in recovery or restorative physiology that occurs overnight.

9. Next, a cascade of recovery hormones initiates the repair, maintenance and rebuilding of bone, muscle and other body tissues. NOTE: For optimized recovery to take place, there must be sufficient glycogen stores in the liver. When liver glycogen stores are adequate, optimized recovery physiology is exclusively fat-burning physiology. Although this seems counterintuitive, the science that documents the burning of fat during rest is well established.

10. Melatonin also impacts memory consolidation by its requirement for the formation of NCAMS – neural cell adhesion molecules – during REM sleep. These are necessary for the processing of short-term memory from the hippocampus into long-term memory in the brain cortex.

11. Concurrent with the above, the fructose moiety of honey carries out its critical role. The liver takes up fructose where it is converted to glucose and stored as liver glycogen, thus providing the brain with a sustained supply of glucose for the night. (Without liver glycogen for fuel, the brain only has sufficient glycogen to survive for about 30 seconds.).

12. Additionally, fructose from honey regulates glucose uptake into the liver by prompting the release of glucokinase from the hepatocyte nuclei. Glucokinase is found primarily in the liver cell nuclei and is necessary for the conversion of glucose to glycogen. This action of fructose in releasing glucokinase is termed in the Honey Diet 'The Fructose Paradox'. Thus, fructose ensures good liver glycogen supply overnight and prevents a major glucose/insulin spike.

13. An adequate liver glycogen supply means that stress hormones (released to maintain fuel supply to the brain in the absence of adequate liver glycogen) need not be released. This exceedingly beneficial effect on an individual's hormone profile over time will have a profound impact on future development of obesity, diabetes and other metabolic conditions.

NOTE: In northern Europe and America, the notion that we should not eat before bedtime results in chronic release of adrenal hormones during the nocturnal fast, impacting sleep architecture and resulting, over time, in increased risk of heart disease, hypertension, osteoporosis, diabetes, obesity, gastric ulcers, childhood obesity, depression, memory loss and dementias – all conditions associated with chronic release of adrenal hormones.

APPENDIX C: WHY HONEY IS THE PERFECT FUEL

Exercise and sleep are two very different metabolic events, but each surprisingly presents the brain with exactly the same challenge – the need for an optimal and continuing energy supply to the brain.

When we exercise, our furiously contracting muscles extract glucose from the circulation at an accelerated rate, rapidly depleting the liver's glycogen stores (which are stockpiled as emergency supplies for the brain).

When we sleep, the same glycogen stores have to keep the brain fuelled until breakfast. If you had supper at 6pm, your poor body might be fasting for as long as 12 hours, and if you skip breakfast, that could be 18 hours.

Whatever happens, the state of the reserve glycogen in the liver determines the timing and intensity of the activation of the HPA (stress) system, which is the only way the brain can ensure a continuing supply of energy.

The timing of the last meal of the day and the size of the liver's glycogen reserve are the key measures that will determine the ability to supply the brain, and the level of activation of the adrenal stress axis. So, if you prefer an early evening meal, it makes simple sense to restock the liver before you go to bed to reduce activation of nocturnal metabolic stress.

If you were going to design a food substance to do the job of restocking the liver's glycogen stores it would need the following characteristics:

1. It should be rapidly absorbed by the gut and put into the circulation, without creating any stress for the digestive system.
2. It should selectively replenish the liver's glycogen reserves without triggering insulin spikes (which would direct any excess into fat reserves).
3. It should stabilize this reserve (Western humans have difficulty forming liver glycogen that stays put, and is only taken up by the brain).
4. It should allow the speedy release of glucose from liver glycogen, as and when required, into the circulation to maintain fuel supply to the brain.
5. It should ensure stable blood glucose levels.
6. It should allow glucose transfer into the brain, even if the mechanism has been suppressed by a high-sugar diet.
7. It should feed the brain and reduce the possibility of brain hunger.
8. In so doing, it should reduce the night-time stress reaction.
9. It should reduce the activation of appetite hormones (which make you crave sweet foods the next day).
10. It should improve the quality and duration of your sleep.
11. It should improve memory and learning during REM sleep.
12. It should improve fat metabolism as the body's recovery processes get to work.

We have no need to design such a food because nature has provided it in the form of honey.

Every night we have the chance to reduce this energy charge, reverse this destructive cycle, and all we have to do is restock the liver just before we go to sleep – with honey.

When honey is the fuel, the extra power is stored in the liver and controlled. We are simply backing up the brain's battery (the liver) and this reserve is released only 'on demand', not subject to the uncontrolled power surges that sugar might cause.

APPENDIX D: HONEY AS A SUPERFOOD

Although each floral source of honey conveys individual profiles in terms of aroma and taste, it seems remarkable (and no co-incidence) that, among the thousands of plant sources of nectar, when transformed into honey all have a similar effect on the absorption, transportation, storage and use (metabolism) of the product, such that a honey produced in Alaska and a honey produced in New Zealand offer exactly the same health benefits. The honey bees produce the same superfood wherever they are located geographically, an outcome that is clearly driven by selective coevolution of the plants and the honey bees, and benefits both.

As well as sugars, honey also contains around two hundred ingredients, each of which is present for a precise reason, and which impart quite amazing dividends to those humans who consume this ancient food.

These consist of vitamins, amino acids, minerals, proteins, bioflavonoids, carotenoids, organic acids, aromatic hydrocarbons, antioxidants, monosaccharides and oligosaccharides, and numerous enzymes including catalase, invertase, glucose oxidase, diastase, phosphatase, and peroxidise. In addition, honey includes two unusual bioactive molecules – hydrogen peroxide and nitric oxide. Many of these important ingredients exert a positive influence on glucose disposal, and therefore on the functioning of the iPump.

In addition, honey stimulates a cascade of beneficial hormones – GLP-1/free IGF-1/leptin. Insulin is stimulated via the HYMN Cycle, promotes melatonin and is then suppressed and controlled via melatonin and growth hormone. This is a beneficial negative feedback mechanism, which happens only during the dark phase of the circadian cycle (at night). No other food can match honey in this respect.

GLP-1 is one of the most beneficial hormones in human metabolism, and is emerging as a key agent of appetite and glycaemic control via a variety of mechanisms. This multi-task hormone exerts a positive influence in the gut/liver/circulation/heart/pancreas/kidney and brain.

NOTES

CHAPTER 1: THE KEY TO WEIGHT LOSS

Dashti HM, al-Zaid NS, Mathew TC, Al-Mousawi M, Talib H, Asfar SK, Behbahani SL. Long-term effects of ketogenic diet in obese subjects with high cholesterol level. Mol Cell Biochem. 2006 Jun;286(1-2):1-9.

Dashti HM, Mathew TC, Khadada M, Al-Mousawi M, Talib H, Asfar SK, Behbahani AL, Al-Zaid NS. Beneficial effects of ketogenic diet in obese diabetic subjects. Mol Cell Biochem. 2007 Aug; 302(1-2):249-56

Freeman JM, Kossof EH, Hartman AL. The ketogenic diet: one decade later. Pediatrics. 2007 Mar;119(3):535-43.

Gardner CD, Kiazand A, Alhassan S, Kim S, Stafford RS, Balise RR, Kraemer HC, Kind AC. Comparison of the Atkins, zone, Ornish and LEARN diets for change in weight and related factors among overweight premenopausal women: the A to Z Weight Loss study: a randomized trial. JAMA. 2007 Mar 7;297(9):969-77.

Gelling RW, Overduin J, Morrison CD, Morton GJ, Frayo RS, Cummings DE, Schwartz MW. Effect of uncontrolled diabetes on plasma ghrelin concentrations and ghrelin-induced feeding. Endocrinology. 2004 Oct;145(10):4575-82.

Harris SC, Ivy AC, Searle LM. The mechanism of amphetamine-induced loss of weight: a consideration of the theory of hunger and appetite. JAMA 1947 Aug 23;134(17):1468-75.

Hite AH, Berkowitz VG, Berkowitz K. Low-carbohydrate diet review: shifting the paradigm. Nutr Clin Pract. 2011 Jun;26(3):300-8.

Hussain TA, Mathew TC, Dashti AA, Asfar S, Al-Zaid N, Dashti HM. Effect of low-calorie versus low-carbohydrate ketogenic diet in type 2 diabetes. Nutrition. 2012 Oct;28(10):1016-21.

The Inuit Paradox. Read how the 75 per cent fat diet of Inuit populations only made them sick and overweight when they introduced refined carbohydrates: http://discovermagazine.com/2004/oct/inuit-paradox#.USOGn-T0CSo

Keys A, Brožek J, Henschel A, Mickelsen O, Taylor H L, (1950). *The Biology of Human Starvation* (2 volumes). St. Paul, MN:University of Minnesota Press MINNE edition.

Kim JE, Kim DS, Kwak SE, Choi HC, Song HK, Choi SY, Kwon OS, Kim YI, Kang TC. Anti-glutamatergic effect of riluzole: comparison with valproic acid. Neuroscience. 2007 Jun 15;147(1):136-45.

Kushner RF, Berman SA. Are high-protein diets effective in McArdle's disease. Arch Neurol. 1090;47(4);382-4.

Dr Robert Lustig is the leading international scientist explaining the role of sugars in modern obesity and an interesting video may be found at: http://www.youtube.com/watch?v=dBnniua6-oM

Mayer J. Regulation of energy intake and the body weight: the glucostatic theory and the lipostatic hypothesis. Ann N Y Acad Sci. 1955 Jul 15;63(1):15-43.

The Mayo Clinic – advice on high-protein diets post-bariatric surgery: http://www.mayoclinic.com/health/gastric-bypass-diet/my00827

Gary Taubes writes about the 'conspiracy' against Robert Atkins: What if it's All Been a Big Fat Lie? *New York Times* Jul 7 2002;

http://www.nytimes.com/2002/07/07/magazine/what-if-it-s-all-been-a-big-fat-lie.html?pagewanted=all&src=pm

Fred Vogelstein's article in the *New York Times Magazine* about his son's epilepsy and how a high-fat diet transformed his life: http://www.nytimes.com/2010/11/21/magazine/21Epilepsy-t.html?pagewanted=all&_r=2&

John Yudkin. *Pure, White and Deadly*. Davis-Poynter Ltd, 1972 (new editions in 1986 and 2012).

Zupec-Kania BA, Spellman E. An overview of the ketogenic diet for pediatric epilepsy. Nutr Clin Pract. 2008 Dec-2009 Jan;23(6):589-96.

An article on UK sugar consumption may be found at: http://www.telegraph.co.uk/health/dietandfitness/9160114/The-bitter-truth-about-sugar.html

Information on sugar consumption in China may be found at: http://www.reuters.com/article/2012/01/18/china-sugar-cba-idUSL3E8C I4LJ20120118

Information on obesity in China may be found at: http://uschina.usc.edu/w_usci/showarticle.aspx?articleID=16595&AspxAutoDetect CookieSupport=1.

CHAPTER 2: SLEEP LIKE A BABY

Awad S, Constantin-Teodosiu D, Constantin D, Rowlans BJ, Fearon KC, Macdonald IA, Lobo DN. Cellular mechanisms underlying the protective effects of preoperative feeding: a randomized study investigating muscle and liver glycogen content, mitochondrial function, gene and protein expression. Ann Surg. 2010 Aug; 252(2):247-53.

Bass J, Turek FW. Sleepless in America: a pathway to obesity and metabolic syndrome? Arch Intern Med. 2005 Jan 10;165(1):15-6.

Bellisle F. Infrequently asked questions about the Mediterranean diet. Public Health Nutr. 2009 Sep;12(9A):1644-7.

Benefice E, Garnier D, Ndiaye G. Nutritional status, growth and sleep habits among Senegalese adolescent girls. Eur J, Clin Nutr. 2004;58:292–301.

Benedict C, Kern W, Schmid SM, Schultes B, Born J. Hallschmid M. Early rise in the hypothalamic-pituitary-adrenal activity: a role for maintaining the brain's energy balance. Psychneuroendocrinology. 2009 Apr;34(3):455-62.

Bullough WS, Eisa EA. The diurnal variations in the tissue glycogen content and their relation to mitotic activity in the adult male mouse. J Exp Biol. 1950 Dec; 27:257.

Cappuccio FP, D'Elia L, Strazzulo P, Miller MA. Sleep duration and all-cause mortality: a systematic review and meta-analysis of prospective studies. Sleep. 2010 May;33(5):585-92.

Center for Disease Control and Prevention – analysis of sleep disorders: http://www.cdc.gov/features/dssleep/

Chaput JP, Brunet M, Tremblay A. Relationship between short sleeping hours and childhood overweight/obesity: results from the 'Quebec en Forme' project. Int J Obes (London). 2006;30:1080-5.

Gangwisch JE, Malaspina D, Boden-Albala B, Heymsfield SB. Inadequate sleep as a risk factor for obesity: analyses of the NHANES I. Sleep. 2005;28:1289-96.

Gupta NK, Mueller WH, Chan W, Meininger JC. Is obesity associated with poor sleep quality in adolescents? Am J Hum Biol. 2002; 14:762-8.

Hasler G, Buysse DJ, Klaghofer R, et al. The association between short sleep duration and obesity in young adults: a 13-year prospective study. Sleep. 2004;27:661-6.

Holden JP, Butzow TL, Laughlin GA, Ho M, Yen SC. Regulation of insulin-like growth factor binding protein-1 during the 24-hour metabolic clock and in response to hypoinsulinaemia induced fasting and Sandostatin in normal women. J Soc Gynecol Invest. 1995 Jan-Feb;2(1):38-44.

Joo EY, Tae WS, Lee MJ, Kang JW, Park HS, Lee JY, Suh M, Hong SB. Reduced brain gray matter concentration in patients with obstructive sleep apnea syndrome. Sleep. 2010 Feb 1;33(2): 235-41.

von Kries R, Toschke AM, Wurmser H, Sauerwald T, Koletzko B. Reduced risk for overweight and obesity in 5- and 6-year-old children by duration of sleep – a cross-sectional study. Int J Obes Relat Metab Disord. 2002;26:710-6.

Knutson KL. Sex differences in the association between sleep and body mass index in adolescents. J Pediatr. 2005;147:830-4.

Ko GT, Chan JC, Chan AW, et al. Association between sleeping hours, working hours and obesity in Hong Kong Chinese: the 'better health for better Hong Kong' health promotion campaign. Int J Obes (London). 2007;31:254-60.

Kohatsu ND, Tsai R, Young T, et al. Sleep duration and body mass index in a rural population. Arch Intern Med. 2006;166:1701-5.

Leproult R, Copinschi G, Buxton O, Van Cauter E. Sleep loss results in elevation of cortisol levels the next evening. Sleep. 1997 Oct;20(10):865-70.

Ljungqvist O, Nygren J, Thorell A. Modulation of post-operative insulin resistance by pre-operative carbohydrate loading. Proc Nutr Soc. 2002 Aug;61(3):329-36.

Moraes W, Azevedo E, Utino A, de Mello M, Tufik S. Weight loss rate during sleep and awake rest. *Journal of Sleep and Sleep Disorders Research*, vol 32 Abstract Supplement. 2009; 23rd annual meeting of the Associated Professional Sleep Societies, LLC Seattle, Washington.

Moreno CR, Louzada FM, Teixeira LR, Borges F, Lorenzi-Filho G. Short sleep is associated with obesity among truck drivers. Chronobiol Int. 2006;23:1295-303.

Naska A, Oikonomou E, Trichopoulou A, Psaltopoulou T, Trichopoulos D. Siesta in healthy adults and coronary mortality in the general population. Arch Intern Med. 2007 Feb 12;167(3):296-301.

Nindl BC, Alemany JA, Tuckow AP, Kellog MD, Sharp MA, Patton JF. Effects of exercise mode and duration on 24-h IGF-1 System recovery responses. Med Sci Sports Exerc. 2009 Jun;41(6):1261-70.

Patel SR, Hu FB. Short sleep duration and weight gain: a systematic review. Obesity (Silver Spring). 2008 Mar; 16(3):643-53.

Pauley SM. Lighting for the human circadian clock: recent research indicates that lighting has become a public health issue. Med Hypotheses. 2004; 63(4):588-96.

Riemann D, Kloepfer C, Berger M. Functional and structural brain alterations in insomnia: implications for pathophysiology. *European Journal of Neuroscience*, vol 29, no 9, May 2009; pp. 1754-60.

Sandercock GR, Voss C, Dye L. Associations between habitual school-day breakfast consumption, body mass index, physical activity and cardiorespiratory fitness in English schoolchildren. Eur J Clin Nutr. 2012 Oct;64(10):1086-92.

Sekine M, Yamagami T, Handa K, et al. A dose-response relationship between short sleeping hours and childhood obesity: results of the Toyama Birth Cohort Study. Child Care Health Dev. 2002;28:163–70.

Singh M, Drake CL, Roehrs T, Hudgel DW, Roth T. The association between obesity and short sleep duration: a population-based study. J Clin Sleep Med. 2005;1:357-63.

Sofer S, Eliraz A, Kaplan S, Voet H, Fink G, Kima T, Madar Z. Greater weight loss and hormonal changes after 6 months diet with carbohydrates eaten mostly at dinner. Obesity (Silver Spring). 2011 Oct;19(10):2006-14.

Spiegel K, Tasali E, Penev P, Van Cauter E. Brief communication: sleep curtailment in healthy young men is associated with decreased leptin levels, elevated ghrelin levels, and increased hunger and appetite. Ann Intern Med. 2004 Dec 7;141(11):846-50.

Vorona RD, Winn MP, Babineau TW, Eng BP, Feldman HR, Ware JC. Overweight and obese patients in a primary care population report less sleep than patients with a normal body mass index. Arch Intern Med. 2005;165:25-30.

Wu YH, Swaab DF. Disturbance and strategies for reactivation of the circadian rhythm system in ageing and Alzheimer's disease. Sleep Med. 2007 Sep;8(6):623-36.

CHAPTER 3: HONEY – THE SWEET MIRACLE

HONEY'S UNEXPECTED QUALITIES

Many studies confirm the health benefits of honey:

1. Cardioprotective activity of honey. By selectively restocking the liver and forward provisioning, the brain honey reduces HPA-driven chronic metabolic stress
2. Antihypertensive activity of honey. Reduction of chronic metabolic stress reduces adrenaline release, and consequent hypertension, particularly overnight
3. Antidiabetic activity in honey is addressed in a study by OO Erejuwa at the University of Malaysia
4. Antioxidant activity of honey is addressed in the same study
5. Honey as an appetite suppressant. A 2010 study at the University of Wyoming found in healthy women that, compared to sucrose, honey reduced ghrelin, an appetite hormone, and upgraded peptide yy, an appetite suppressant
6. Honey protects the brain (because it keeps the brain's feeder cells well stocked with fuel)
7. Honey for weight control. In 2009, a group at the Medical Sciences/University of Tehran found that honey had a positive influence on weight control and lipids in diabetic patients who took honey and not on those who did not, over an 8-week period. Honey is known to be a potent antioxidant and antioxidant activity appears to contribute to weight control by improving insulin sensitivity (something other sugars don't do). An emerging field of study, led by

Wayne Lautt at the University of Manitoba, is in post-meal insulin sensitivity. It is beginning to show that antioxidant potential reduces both hyperglycaemia and hyperinsulinism, with a positive impact on weight control and diabetes

8. Honey can boost your memory. Although no studies (so far) have directly demonstrated that honey may exert a positive influence on memory and learning, it does aid sleep, and quality sleep is the optimum period for consolidation of memories. In addition, honey promotes a cascade of nocturnal hormones that recalibrate and facilitate the cerebral glucose pump – the iPump – creating the perfect nocturnal metabolic environment for improved cognition and learning. A recent review (by Rasch and Born, below) distinguished between sleep (a time for memory consolidation) and being awake (a time for encoding information). The authors emphasize that memory hippocampus and immune memory are consolidated during sleep. They say: 'Over more than a century of research has established the fact that *sleep* benefits the retention of *memory* . . . While elaborated with respect to hippocampus-dependent memories, the concept of an active redistribution of *memory* representations from networks serving as temporary store into long-term stores might hold also for non-hippocampus-dependent memory, and even for non-neuronal, i.e., immunological memories, giving rise to the idea that the offline consolidation of *memory* during *sleep* represents a principle of long-term *memory* formation established in quite different physiological systems'

9. Honey protects the gut. In 1999, a group at the Baylor College of Medicine and the Veterans Affairs Medical Center in Houston, Texas, examined the effect of honey on the growth of *H. pylori* in vitro. They found both hydrogen peroxide and

non hydrogen peroxide killing mechanisms, and identified osmosis as one of the key mechanisms for honey inhibition of *H. pylori*

10. Honey has a positive role in liver function. A 2003 study on sheep using intravenous and intrapulmonary administration of honey showed a positive influence on blood sugar concentrations, on lipid profile, bone marrow function and in carbon tetrachloride-induced liver function: 'Results showed that IV or *intrapulmonary administration* of *honey* did not cause any adverse effect. *Intravenous* delivery of honey by slow infusion caused improvement of *renal* and hepatic *function, bone marrow function,* and *lipid profile*'

11. Honey is antibacterial. A 2012 Canadian study at Brock University in Ontario demonstrated inhibition of growth in two highly resistant organisms – MRSA (methicillin-resistant *Staphylococcus aureus*) and VRE (vancomycin-resistant *Enterococcus faecium*). 'We have demonstrated for the first time that bacteriostatic effect of honeys on *MRSA* and VRE was dose-dependently related to generation of (•)OH from *honey* H(2)O(2)'

12. In 1996, a study at the Tashreen Hospital in Damascus examined the potential of honey to inhibit the rubella virus: 'Our results indicated that *honey* had good anti-*rubella* activity'

13. In 2011, a study at the University of Santiago de Compostela, in Spain, tested honey for antifungal activity and found that fungal organisms were inhibited. Honey samples tested on *Candida albicans, Candida krusei,* and *Cryptococcus neoformans* showed, 'growth of all the yeasts was reduced in the presence of *honey*'

14. A 2010 study at the University of Malaysia and published in the journal *Nutritional Research* found potent anti-inflammatory activity in honey extracts containing varying amounts of

> phenolic compounds – the major ones being: *ellagic*, gallic, and
> ferulic *acids*; myricetin; chlorogenic *acid*; and caffeic *acid*
>
> 15. In 2010, a Japanese study at Kyoto Sangyo University examined
>   jungle honey sourced by wild honey bees in Nigeria and found
>   it possessed 'potent antitumour activity'

These and other studies demonstrate that science has recently woken up to the medical potential of honey beyond its topical anti-infective potential.

Abdulrhman M, El-Hefnawy M, Hussein R, et al. The glycemic and peak incremental indices of honey, sucrose and glucose in patients with type 1 diabetes mellitus: effects on C-peptide level – a pilot study. Acta Diabetol. 2011;48:89-94.

Abdulrhman M, El-Hefnawy M, Ali R, et al. Honey and type 1 diabetes mellitus. In: (ed.) Liu CP. Type 1 diabetes – complications, pathogenesis, and alternative treatments. Croatia: InTech. 2011:228-33.

Agrawal OP, Pachauri A, Yadav H, et al. Subjects with impaired glucose tolerance exhibit a high degree of tolerance to honey. J Med Food. 2007;10:473-8.

Ahmad A, Azim MK, Mesaik MA. Natural honey modulates physiological response compared to simulated honey and D-glucose. J Food Sci. 2008;73:H165-7.

Ahmed A, Khan RA, Azim MK, et al. Effect of natural honey on human platelets and blood coagulation proteins. Pak J Pharm Sci. 2011;24:389-97.

Al-Waili NS. Natural honey lowers plasma glucose, C-reactive protein, homocysteine, and blood lipids in healthy, diabetic, and hyperlipidemic subjects: comparison with dextrose and sucrose. J Med Food. 2004;7:100-7.

Al-Waili NS. Intrapulmonary administration of natural honey solution, hyperosmolar dextrose or hypoosmolar distill water to normal individuals and to patients with type 2 diabetes mellitus or hypertension: their effects on blood glucose level, plasma insulin and C-peptide, blood pressure and peaked expiratory flow rate. Eur J Med Res. 2003;8:295-303.

Al-Waili NS. Intravenous and intrapulmonary administration of honey solution to healthy sheep: effects on blood sugar, renal and liver function tests, bone marrow function, lipid profile, and carbon tetrachloride-induced liver injury. J Med Food. 2003;6:231-47.

Al-Waili NS. Effects of daily consumption of honey solution on hematological indices and blood levels of minerals and enzymes in normal individuals. J Med Food. 2003;6:135-40.

Al-Waili NS. Effects of honey on the urinary total nitrite and prostaglandins concentration. Int Urol Nephrol. 2005;37:107-11.

Arnon SS, Midura TF, Damus K, et al. Honey and other environmental risk factors for infant botulism. J Pediatr. 1979;94:331-6.

Bahrami M, Ataie-Jafari A, Hosseini S, Foruzanfar MH, Rahmani M, Pajouhi M. Effects of natural honey consumption in diabetic patients: an 8-week randomized clinical trial. Int J Food Sci Nutr. 2009;60:618-26.

Boehme MW, Autschbach F, Ell C, et al. Prevalence of silent gastric ulcer, erosions or severe acute gastritis in patients with type 2 diabetes mellitus – a cross-sectional study. Hepatogastroenterology. 2007;54:643-8.

Bogdanov S. Honey as nutrient and functional food. http://www.bee-hexagon.net

Brudaynski K, Lannigan R. Mechanism of honey bactriostatic action against MRSA and VRE involves hydrogen radicals generated from honey's hydrogen peroxide. Front Microbiol. 2012;3:36.

Busserolles J, Gueux E, Rock E, et al. Substituting honey for refined carbohydrates protects rats from hypertriglyceridemic and prooxidative effects of fructose. J Nutr. 2002;132:3379-82.

Cani PD, Neyrinck AM, Fava F, et al. Selective increases of bifidobacteria in gut microflora improve high-fat-diet-induced diabetes in mice through a mechanism associated with endotoxaemia. Diabetologia. 2007;50:2374-83.

Chepulis LM, Starkey N. The long-term effects of feeding honey compared with sucrose and a sugar-free diet on weight gain, lipid profiles, and DEXA measurements in rats. J Food Sci. 2008;73:H1-7.

Chepulis LM. The effect of honey compared to sucrose, mixed sugars, and a sugar-free diet on weight gain in young rats. J Food Sci. 2007;72:S224-9.

Ciudad CJ, Carabaza A, Guinovart JJ. Glycogen synthesis from glucose and fructose in hepatocytes from diabetic rats. Arch Biochem Biophys. 1988;267:437-47.

Crane E. History of honey. In: (ed.) Crane E. *Honey, a comprehensive survey*. London: William Heinemann. 1975:439-88.

Eraslan G, Kanbur M, Silici S, et al. Beneficial effect of pine honey on trichlorfon induced some biochemical alterations in mice. Ecotoxicol Environ Saf. 2010;73:1084-91.

Erejuwa OO, Sulaiman SA, Wahab MSA. Honey – a novel antidiabetic agent. Int J Biol Sci. 2012;8(6):913-34. doi:10.7150/ijbs.3697.

Erejuwa OO. The use of honey in diabetes mellitus: is it beneficial or detrimental? Int J Endocrinol Metab. 2012;10:444-5.

Erejuwa OO, Sulaiman SA, Wahab MS, et al. Comparison of anti-oxidant effects of honey, glibenclamide, metformin, and their combinations in the kidneys of streptozotocin-induced diabetic rats. Int J Mol Sci. 2011;12:829-43.

Erejuwa OO, Sulaiman SA, Wahab MS, et al. Glibenclamide or metformin combined with honey improves glycemic control in streptozotocin-induced diabetic rats. Int J Biol Sci. 2011;7:244-52.

Erejuwa OO, Sulaiman SA, Wahab MS, et al. Hepatoprotective effect of tualang honey supplementation in streptozotocin-induced diabetic rats. Int J Appl Res Nat Prod. 2012;4:37-41.

Erejuwa OO, Gurtu S, Sulaiman SA, et al. Hypoglycemic and

antioxidant effects of honey supplementation in streptozotocin-induced diabetic rats. Int J Vitam Nutr Res. 2010;80:74-82.

Erejuwa OO, Sulaiman SA, Wahab MS, et al. Antioxidant protective effect of glibenclamide and metformin in combination with honey in pancreas of streptozotocin-induced diabetic rats. Int J Mol Sci. 2010;11:2056-66.

Erejuwa OO, Sulaiman SA, Wahab MS, et al. Antioxidant protection of Malaysian tualang honey in pancreas of normal and streptozotocin-induced diabetic rats. Ann Endocrinol (Paris). 2010;71:291-6.

Erejuwa OO, Sulaiman SA, Wahab MS, et al. Honey supplementation in spontaneously hypertensive rats elicits antihypertensive effect via amelioration of renal oxidative stress. Oxid Med Cell Longev. 2012;2012:1-14.

Erejuwa OO, Sulaiman SA, Wahab MS, Fructose might contribute to the hypoglycemic effect of honey. Molecules. 2012;17:1900-15.

Erejuwa OO, Sulaiman SA, Wahab MS, et al. Effects of Malaysian tualang honey supplementation on glycemia, free radical scavenging enzymes and markers of oxidative stress in kidneys of normal and streptozotocin-induced diabetic rats. Int J Cardiol. 2009;137:S45.

Erejuwa OO, Sulaiman SA, Wahab MS, et al. Effect of glibenclamide alone versus glibenclamide and honey on oxidative stress in pancreas of streptozotocin-induced diabetic rats. Int J Appl Res Nat Prod. 2011;4:1-10.

Erejuwa OO, Sulaiman SA, Wahab MS, et al. Differential responses to blood pressure and oxidative stress in streptozotocin-induced diabetic wistar-kyoto rats and spontaneously hypertensive rats: effects of antioxidant (honey) treatment. Int J Mol Sci. 2011;12:1888-907.

Erejuwa OO, Sulaiman SA, Wahab MS. Honey: a novel antioxidant. Molecules. 2012;17:4400-23.

Erejuwa OO, Sulaiman SA, Wahab MS, et al. Influence of rat strains and/or severity of hyperglycemia on systolic blood pressure and antioxidant enzymes in kidney of rats with hypertension and/or diabetes: role of honey. Int J Cardiol. 2011;152:S29.

Ergul E, Ergul S. The effect of honey on the intestinal anastomotic wound healing in rats with obstructive jaundice. World J Gastroenterol. 2008;14:3410-5.

Fasanmade AA, Alabi OT. Differential effect of honey on selected variables in alloxan-induced and fructose-induced diabetic rats. Afr J Biomed Res. 2008;11:191-6.

Feas X, Estevinho ML. A survey of the in vitro antifungal activity of heather (Erica sp.) organic honey. J Med Food. 2011;14:1284-8.

Fukuda M, Kobayashi K, Hirono Y, et al. Jungle honey enhances immune function and antitumour activity. Evid Based Complement Alternat Med. 2011;2011:1-8.

Gencay C, Kilicoglu SS, Kismet K, et al. Effect of honey on bacterial translocation and intestinal morphology in obstructive jaundice. World J Gastroenterol. 2008;14:3410-5.

Gharzhouli K, Amira S, Gharzouli A, et al. Gastroprotective effects of honey and glucose-fructose-sucrose-maltose mixture against ethanol-, indomethacin-, and acidified aspirin-induced lesions in the rat. Exp Toxicol Pathol. 2002;54:217-21.

Gheldof N, Wang XH, Engeseth NJ. Buckwheat honey increases serum antioxidant capacity in humans. J Agric Food Chem. 2003; 51:1500-5.

Gheldof N, Engeseth NJ. Antioxidant capacity of honeys from various floral sources based on the determination of oxygen radical absorbance capacity and inhibition of in vitro lipoprotein oxidation in human serum samples. J Agric Food Chem. 2002;50:3050-5.

Gollu A, Kismet K, Kilicoglu B, et al. Effect of honey on intestinal morphology, intra-abdominal adhesions and anastomotic healing. Phytother Res. 2008;22:1243-7.

Honey bee immunity and refined sugars: http://science.nbcnews.com/_news/2013/04/29/17974455-best-rx-for-bees-their-own-honey?lite

Honey bee feeding: http://science.nbcnews.com/_news/2013/04/29/ 17974455-best-rx-for-bees-their-own-honey?lite

Jones HF, Butler RN, Brooks DA. Intestinal fructose transport and malabsorption in humans. Am J Physiol Gastrointest Liver Physiol. 2011;300:G202-6.

Jorgensen JOL, Larsen RL, Moller L, Krag M, Jessen N, Norrelund H, Christiansen JS, Moller N. Growth hormone and insulin resistance. *Hormone Research* vol 67, suppl. 1,2007.

Kabadi UM. Is hepatic glycogen content a regulator of glucagon secretion? Metabolism. 1992 Feb;41(2):113-5.

Kammer AE, Heinrich B. Insect flight metabolism. Adv. Insect Physiol. 1978;13:133-228. Foraging honey bees can increase their metabolic rate from rest to flight by a factor of 70.

Kassim M, Achoui M, Mustafa MR, et al. Ellagic acid, phenolic acids, and flavonoids in Malaysian honey extracts demonstrate in vitro anti-inflammatory activity. Nutr Res. 2010;30:650-9.

Katsilambros NL, Philippides P, Touliatou A, et al. Metabolic effects of honey (alone or combined with other foods) in type 2 diabetics. Acta Diabetol Lat. 1988;25:197-203.

Khalil MI, Alam N, Moniruzzaman M, et al. Phenolic acid composition and antioxidant properties of Malaysian honeys. J Food Sci. 2011;76:C921-8.

Kishore RK, Halim AS, Syazana MS,. et al. Tualang honey has higher phenolic content and greater radical scavenging activity compared with other honey sources. Nutr Res. 2011;31:322-5.

Koca I, Koca AF. Poisoning by mad honey: a brief review. Food Chem Toxicol. 2007;45:1315-8.

Larson-Meyer DE, Willis KS, Willis LM, et al. Effect of honey versus sucrose on appetite, appetite-regulating hormones, and postmeal thermogenesis. J Am Coll Nutr. 2010;29:482-93.

Lautt WW, Ming Z, Legare DJ. Attenuation of age- and sucrose-induced insulin resistance and syndrome X by a synergistic antioxidant cocktail: the AMIS syndrome and HISS hypothesis. Can J Physiol Pharmacol. 2010 Mar;88(3):313-23.

Lavin JH, Wittert GA, Andrews J, et al. Interaction of insulin, glucagon-like peptide 1, gastric inhibitory polypeptide, and appetite in response to intraduodenal carbohydrate. Am J Clin Nutr. 1998;68:591-8.

Lee SO, Choi SZ, Lee JH, Chung SH, Park SH, Kang HC, Yang EY, Cho HJ, Lee KR. Antidiabetic coumarin and cyclitol compounds from *Peucedanum japonicum*. Arch Pharm Res. 2004 Dec;27(12):1207-10.

Madero M, Arriaga JC, Jalal D, et al. The effect of two energy-restricted diets, a low-fructose diet versus a moderate natural fructose diet, on weight loss and metabolic syndrome parameters: a randomized controlled trial. Metabolism. 2011;60:1551-9.

Mao W, Schuler MA, Berenbaum MR. Honey constituents up-regulate detoxification and immunity genes in the Western honey bee *Apis mellifera*. Proc Natl Acad Sci USA. 2013 Apr 29 (ahead of print).

Mohamed M, Sirajudeen K, Swamy M, et al. Studies on the antioxidant properties of Tualang honey of Malaysia. Afr J Tradit Complement Altern Med. 2010;7:59-63.

Moran TH, McHugh PR. Distinctions among three sugars in their effects on gastric emptying and satiety. Am J Physiol. 1981;241:R25-30.

Munstedt K, Sheybani B, Hauenschild A, et al. Effects of basswood honey, honey-comparable glucose-fructose solution, and oral glucose tolerance test solution on serum insulin, glucose, and C-peptide concentrations in healthy subjects. J Med Food. 2008;11:424-8.

Munstedt K, Hoffmann S, Hauenschild A, et al. Effect of honey on serum cholesterol and lipid values. J Med Food. 2009;12:624-8.

Nemoseck TM, Carmody EG, Furchner-Evanson A, et al. Honey promotes lower weight gain, adiposity, and triglycerides than sucrose in rats. Nutr Res. 2011;31:55-60.

Osato MS, Reddy SG, Graham DY. Osmotic effect of honey on growth and viability of *Helicobacter pylori*. Dig Dis Sci. 1999;44:462-4.

Paul IM, Beiler J, McMonagle A, Schaffer ML, Duda L, Berlin CM Jr. Effect of honey, dextromethorpan, and no treatment on nocturnal cough and sleep quality for coughing children and their parents. Arch Pediatr Adolesc Med. 2007 Dec;161(12):1140-6.

Rakha MK, Nabil ZI, Hussein AA. Cardioactive and vasoactive effects of natural wild honey against cardiac malperformance induced by hyperadrenergic activity. J Med Food. 2008;11:91-8.

Regan JJ Jr, Doorneweerd DD, Gilboe DP, Nuttall FQ. Influence of fructose on the glycogen synthase and phosphorylase systems in rat liver metabolism. 1980;29:965-9.

Robert SD, Ismail AA. Two varieties of honey that are available in Malaysia gave intermediate glycemic index values when tested among healthy individuals. Biomed Pap Med Fac Univ Palacky Olomouc Czech Repub. 2009;153:145-7.

Samanta A, Burden AC, Jones GR. Plasma glucose responses to glucose, sucrose, and honey in patients with diabetes mellitus: an analysis of glycemic and peak incremental indices. Diabet Med. 1985;2:371-3.

Shambaugh P, Worthington V, Herbert JH. Differential effects of honey, sucrose, and fructose on blood sugar levels. J Manipulative Physiol Ther. 1990;13:322-5.

Shin HS, Ustunol Z. Carbohydrate composition of honey from different floral sources and their influence on growth of selected intestinal bacteria: an in vitro comparison. Food Res Int. 2005;38:721-8.

Shiota M, Galasseti P, Igawa K. Inclusion of low amounts of fructose with an intraportal glucose load increases net hepatic glucose uptake in the presence of insulin deficiency in dog. Am J Physiol Endocrinol Metab. 2005;288:E1160-7.

Tan HT, Rahman RA, Gan SH, et al. The antibacterial properties of Malaysian tualang honey against wound and enteric microorganisms in comparison to Manuka honey. BMC Complement Altern Med. 2009;9:1-8.

Tanzi MG, Gabay MP. Association between honey consumption and infant botulism. Pharmacotherapy. 2002;22:1479-83.

Vaisman N, Niv E, Izkhakov Y. Catalytic amounts of fructose may improve glucose tolerance in subjects with uncontrolled non-insulin-dependent diabetes. Clin Nutr. 2006;25:617-21.

Valcavi R, Zini M, Maestroni GJ, Conti A, Portioli I. Melatonin stimulates growth hormone secretion through pathways other than the growth hormone releasing hormone. Clin Endocrinol (Oxford). 1993 Aug;39(2):193-9.

Van Schaftingen E, Davies DR. Fructose administration stimulates glucose phosphorylation in the livers of anaesthetized rats. FASEB J. 1991;5:326-30.

Wang J, Li QX. Chemical composition, characterization, and differentiation of honey botanical and geographical origins. Adv Food Nutr Res. 2011;62:89-137.

Watford M. Small amounts of dietary fructose dramatically increase hepatic glucose uptake through a novel mechanism of glucokinase activation. Nutr Rev. 2002;60:253-7.

Wei Y, Bizeau ME, Pagliassotti MJ. An acute increase in fructose concentration increases hepatic glucose-6-phosphatase mRNA via mechanisms that are independent of glycogen synthase kinase-3 in rats. J Nutr. 2004;134:545-51.

Yaghoobi N, Al-Waili NS, Ghayour-Mobarhan M, et al. Natural honey and cardiovascular risk factors; effects on blood glucose, cholesterol, triacylglycerole, CRP, and body weight compared with sucrose. Scientific World Journal. 2008;8:463-9.

Young JH, Kaslow HR, Bergman RN. Fructose effect to suppress hepatic glycogen degradation. J Biol Chem. 1987;262:11470-7.

Zeina B, Othman O, al-Assad S. Effect of honey versus thyme on rubella virus survival in vitro. J Altern Complement Med. 1996; 2:345-8.

CHAPTER 7: BOOST YOUR BRAIN POWER

Aiello Leslie C, Wheeler P. The expensive-tissue hypothesis: the brain and the digestive system in human and primate evolution. *Current Anthropology*, vol 36, no2, Apr 1995; pp. 199-221.

Baker LD, Cross DJ, Minoshima S, Belongia D, Watson GS, Craft S. Insulin resistance and Alzheimer's-like reductions in regional cerebral glucose metabolism for cognitively normal adults with prediabetes or early type 2 diabetes. Arch Neurol. 2011 Jan;68(1):51-7.

Bruehl H, Sweat V, Tirsi A, Shah B, Convit A. Obese adolescents with type 2 diabetes mellitus have hippocampal and front lobe volume reductions. Neurosci Med. 2011 Mar 1:2(1):34-42.

Castellanos FX, Lee PP, Sharp W, Jeffries NO, Greenstein DK, Clasen LS, Blumenthal JD, James RS, Ebens CL, Walter JM, Zijdenbos A, Evans AC, Giedd JN, Rapoport JL: Developmental trajectories of brain volume abnormalities in children and adolescents with attention-deficit/hyperactivity disorder. JAMA., 2002, 288:1740-8.

Cornier MA, McFadden KL, Thomas EA, Bechtell Jl, Eichman LS, Bessesen DH, Tegellas JR. Differences in the neuronal response to food in obesity-resistant as compared to obesity-prone individuals. Physiol Behav. 2013 Feb 17;110-111:122-8.

Delvenne V, Goldman S, De Maertelaar V, Lotstra F. Brain glucose metabolism in eating disorders assessed by positron emission tomography. Int J Eat Disord. 1999 Jan;25(1):29-37.

Excellent article by Professor Marian C Diamond who measured glia/neurone ratios in Einstein's brain: http://education.jhu.edu/PD/newhorizons/Neurosciences/articles/einstein/

Diamond MC, Scheibel AB, Murphy GM, Murphy GM Jr, Harvey T. On the brain of a scientist: Albert Einstein. Exp Neurol. 1985 Apr;88(1):198-204.

Durston S, Hulshoff Pol HE, Schnack HG, Buitelaar JK, Steenhuis MP, Minderaa RB, Kahn RS, van EH: Magnetic resonance imaging of boys with attention-deficit/hyperactivity disorder and their unaffected siblings. J Am Acad Child Adolesc Psychiatry. 2004; 43:332-40.

Ernst M, Zametkin AJ, Matochik J, Schmidt M, Jons PH, Liebenauer LL, Hardy KK, Cohen RM. Intravenous dextroamphetamine and brain glucose metabolism. Neuropsychopharmacology. 1997 Dec; 17(6):391-401.

Filipek PA, Semrud-Clikeman M, Steingard RJ, Renshaw PF, Kennedy DN, Biederman J: Volumetric MRI analysis comparing subjects having attention-deficit hyperactivity disorder with normal controls. Neurology. 1997; 48:589-601.

Fowler SP, Williams J, Esendez RG, Hunt KJ, Hazuda HP, Stern MP. Fuelling the obesity epidemic? Artificially sweetened beverage use and long-term weight gain. Obesity (Silver Spring). 2008 Aug; 16(8): 1894-900.

Grunstein HS, James DE, Storlien LH, Smythe GA, Kraegen EW. Hyperinsulinemia suppresses glucose utilization in specific brain regions: in vivo studies using the euglycemic clamp in the rat. Endocrinology. 1985 Feb;116(2):604-10.

Lim SK, Park MJ, Lim JC, Kim JC, Han HJ, Kim GY, Cravatt BF, Woo Ch, Ma SJ, Yoon KC, Park SH. Hyperglycemia induces apoptosis via CB! activation through the decrease of FAAH 1 in retinal pigment epithelial cells. J Cell Physiol. 2012 Feb;227(2):569-77.

McCall AL, Millington WR, Wurtman RJ. Metabolic fuel and amino acid transport into the brain in experimental diabetes. Proc Natl Acad Sci USA. 1982 Sept;79(17):5406-10.

Magistretti PJ, Pellerin L. Cellular mechanisms of brain energy metabolism and their relevance to functional brain imaging. Philos Trans R Soc Lond B Biol Sci. 1999 Jul 29;354(1387):1153-63.

Meijssen S, Cabezas MC, Ballieux CG, Derksen RJ, Bilecen S, Erklens DW. Insulin mediated inhibition of hormone sensitive lipase activity in vivo in relation to endogenous catecholamines in healthy subjects. J Clin Endocrinol Metab. 2001 Sep;86(9):4193-7.

Mostofsky SH, Cooper KL, Kates WR, Denckla MB, Kaufman WE. Smaller prefrontal and premotor volumes in boys with attention-deficit/hyperactivity disorder. Biol Psychiatry. 2002 Oct 15;52(80:785-94. 'Boys with ADHD had (on average) 8.3% smaller total cerebral volumes. Significant reductions in lobar volumes were seen only for the frontal lobes. Within the frontal lobes, a reduction was seen in both gray and white matter volumes, with some evidence suggesting lateralization of these findings: reduction in frontal white matter volume was specific to the left hemisphere; there was a bilateral reduction in frontal gray matter volume but more so in the right hemisphere. Subparcellation of the frontal lobe revealed smaller prefrontal, premotor, and deep white matter volumes.'

Ola MS, Hosoya K, LaNoue KF. Influence of insulin on glutamine synthetase in the Muller glial cells of the retina. Metab Brain Dis. 2011 Sep;26(3):195-202.

Peters A. The selfish brain: competition for energy resources. Am J Hum Biol. 2011 Jan-Feb; 23(1):29-34.

Raji CA, Ho AJ, Parikshak NN, Becker JT, Lopez OL, Kuller LH, Hua X, Leow AD, Toga AW, Thompson PM. Hum Brain Mapp. 2010 Mar;31(3):353-64. 'Higher BMI was associated with lower brain volumes in overweight and obese elderly subjects. Obesity is therefore associated with detectable brain volume deficits in cognitively normal elderly subjects.'

Reser JE. Alzheimer's disease and natural cognitive ageing may represent adaptive metabolism reduction programs. Behav Brain Funct. 2009 Feb 28;5:13.

Ros S, Garcia-Rocha M, Calbo J, Guinovart JJ. Restoration of hepatic glycogen deposition reduces hyperglycaemia, hyperphagia and gluconeogenic enzymes in a streptozotocin-induced model of diabetes in rats. Diabetologia. 2011 Oct;54(10):2639-48.

Russel VA, Oades RD, Tannock R, Killeen PR, Auerbach JG, Johansen EB, Sagvolden T. Response variability in attention-deficit/hyperactivity disorder: a neuronal and glial energetic hypothesis. Behav Brain Function. 2006 Aug 23;2:30.

Salehi A, Vieira E, Gylfe E. Paradoxical stimulation of glucagon secretion by high glucose concentrations. Diabetes. 2006 Aug;55(8):2318-23.

Swithers SE, Davidson TL. A role for sweet taste: calorie predictive relations in energy regulation by rats. Behav Neurosci. 2008 Feb;122(1):161-73.

Tadjore M, Bergeron R, Latour M, Desy F, Warren C, Lavoie J-M. Effects of dietary manipulations and glucose infusion on glucagon response during exercise in rats. J Appl Physiol. 1997 Jul;83(1):148-52.

Tirsi A, Duong M, Tsui W, Lee C, Convit A. Retinal vessel abnormalities as a possible biomarker of brain volume loss in obese adolescents. Obesity (Silver Spring). 2013 Mar 20. Doi: 10. 1002/oby. 20450. Epub ahead of print.

Todd RD, Boteron KN. Is attention-deficit/hyperactivity disorder an energy deficiency syndrome? Biol Psychiatry. 2001 Aug 1;50(3):151-8.

Yau PL, Castro MG, Tagani A, Tsui WH, Convit A. Obesity and metabolic syndrome and functional and structural brain impairments in adolescents. Pediatrics. 2012 Oct;130(4):e856-6.

Yost TJ, Jensen DR, Haugen BR, Eckel RH. Effect of dietary macronutrient composition on tissue-specific lipoprotein lipase activity in normal-weight subjects. Am J Clin Nutr. 1998 Aug;68(2):296-302.

ABOUT THE AUTHOR

Mike McInnes was born in Edinburgh in 1943, he attended Holy Cross Academy and then went on to study pharmacy at Heriot-Watt College, qualifying as a pharmacist in 1969. After working as a pharmacist for Boots and in private practice, he finally opened his own pharmacy in the Craigentinny/Lochend area of Edinburgh in 1983. In the 1990s, Mike commissioned John Dewar of the architects Dignan Read and Dewar to build a radical new modernist pharmacy in steel and glass. In 1994 this new pharmacy won first prize in the most prestigious Scottish architectural award, The Regeneration of Scotland Award, and became one of the most successful community pharmacies in Scotland. In 1997, Mike sold his pharmacy to The Boots Company.

From this point Mike then focussed his attention on sports nutrition, researching the specifics of energy partition and selection during exercise.

His research led him to believe that honey could be the Gold Standard fuel for forward provisioning the brain, via the liver, during exercise and stocking up for recovery. Further research resulted in the discovery that sleep is a high-energy system with respect to the brain, and that failure to forward provision the brain prior to sleep leads to chronic nocturnal metabolic stress and aborted recovery.

He continues his studies into the health benefits of honey, and is passionately convinced that the Honey Diet could be the most significant and cost-effective contribution to public health and learning in several generations.

Mike lives in Edinburgh with his wife Theresa. They have four children: Christine, Stuart, Graham and Janet and three grand-children: Oskar, Rob and Isla, all of whom love honey.

ACKNOWLEDGEMENTS

I would like to thank Louise Atkinson for converting my convoluted and turgid prose into English, and her husband Jonathan Woods for his beautiful depiction of the iPump, the suppression of which drives obesity/diabetes and Alzheimer's disease in addition to a wide range of both physiological and neurological diseases.

Many thanks also to my agent Robin Wade, and my editor Mark Booth for recognising the potential of my research and hypotheses in combating the above conditions.

Thanks also to my son Stuart for early discussions on liver glycogen metabolism, to Tim Dew whose intellectual support and advice has been invaluable, to Alex Dunedin, the founder of the wonderful Ragged University, for countless and fruitful discussions on impaired energy metabolism, and to David Elliott for his valued support and for guiding me to relevant studies that I missed.